THE CANCER RISK

NOBODY DARES TO TALK ABOUT

BY BRUNO BARMUS

Published by: Fact Publishing
Post Office Box 26B42
Los Angeles, CA 90026, U.S.A.

Library of Congress Catalog Card Number 84-90314

ISBN 0-9613171-0-8

First Printing: 1984

Printed in the United States of America

Cover Design: Peter M. Barmus

About the Author

BRUNO BARMUS was born and educated in Europe, where he taught physical education and related health science.

In 1951, he emigrated to the United States of America. This book, his first, is the result of extensive research he conducted in response to concerns about certain medical and dental procedures in this country that, he feels, pose serious health risks to the public. He endeavored to break through the self-protecting apparatus of the medical and dental establishments in search of answers to his serious inquiries. He questioned government regulations over medical practices, enacted without enforcement provisions. He believes that the medical and dental establishments have within their power the ability to substantially diminish the cancer risk to us all, but that it is not in their best interest to do so, nor is it in the best interest of other related industries. These shocking conclusions are drawn from a meticulous examination of the facts.

Acknowledgment

For criticism and assistance in the preparation of this manuscript I am indebted to my wife, Ursula Barmus, my son Peter, and editor Loretta Rooney Hess.

TABLE OF CONTENTS

PREFACE

Why are more and more Americans suffering from cancer? What are the sources of the danger? The sun gets blamed for skin cancer. Smoking is blamed for lung cancer. And now the latest cancer research is directed toward the risks from natural food toxins. We are told that our diet represents a major factor in cancer, second only to tobacco smoking, which is said to cause 30 percent of all cancer deaths.

Yet little, if anything, is being said about the dangers of needless overexposure to x-rays. Close to one billion medical and dental x-ray films are taken annually in the United States. At least 30 percent of those are unnecessary, according to several official sources. Even more significant is the fact that radiation doses for the same x-ray procedure vary dramatically, instead of being a standard amount. The variations depend on the facility, the age and condition of the x-ray unit involved, and the expertise of those who operate the units. A substandard or improperly adjusted machine may be dangerously overexposing a consumer who is unaware of the risk. Of the machines in use today, 80% were built before manufacturing standards were established, and there are no controls over their performance. This represents a serious health hazard yet to be dealt with in cancer research.

The consumer is uninformed about possible x-ray overexposure dangers; and if he does raise questions, he is quickly reassured that x-ray equipment has been considerably improved and x-radiation exposure doses are minimal and hardly of concern. My research has shown that nothing could be further from the truth.

With this book, I am trying to expose the fallacy of those claims and hoping to instigate desperately-needed legislative reforms for proper consumer protection from dangerous, cancer-causing radiation overexposure.

Present laws provide for inspection of machines. But this is meaningless without legislation to regulate use and correct deficiencies. So far, the medical and dental lobbies have prevented the passage of such laws. I am appealing to lawmakers and professionals alike to join in taking the necessary steps: limit to the absolute minimum the number of x-rays to be taken; mandate licensing of x-ray machine operators; and, most important, prohibit the use of substandard x-ray machines with high exposure levels in dental and medical facilities.

I.

X-RAYS:
FACT, DANGER, AND MYTH

Consumers and practitioners alike depend on existing radiation control laws for their protection. It is a naive and dangerous dependence. The time has come to question the effectiveness of these laws, to point out their flaws and omissions, and to ask why these are not being corrected.

All the evidence points to a link between cancer and x-radiation. The increase in breast cancer incidence, for example, has occurred during the same years breast x-ray examinations have become routine. Instead of researching this curious coincidence, however, health professionals continue to advise women through the news media to undergo *more* breast x-ray examinations to detect the presence of cancer. This is analogous to the inducement of adverse health effects for the sake of detection.

Nevertheless, x-ray machines are widely used in medical and dental offices. In many cases, patients are casually — almost thoughtlessly — subjected to x-ray examinations by doctors, administrators, and insurers, with the simple explanation that the diagnostic x-radiation exposure is negligible and there is nothing to worry about. My long, arduous investigation revealed different, shocking facts. I found that x-ray dosage for the same procedure varies dramatically among different facilities, which points to the widespread use of substandard x-ray equipment and the practice of allowing untrained personnel to operate x-ray machines.

It is not generally understood by the public that substandard equipment is still in use, because the law fails to require updating to safer standards any machine made before 1974. The federal standard applies to major components as well as complete systems made *after* August 1, 1974. The manufacturer determines how to achieve levels of equipment performance set by the standard. Certification by the manufacturer is required to show compliance with federal provisions.

Consumers have been lulled into believing the law protects them. After all, the Federal Radiation Control for Health and Safety Act was enacted in 1968, more than 15 years ago. At the time of its enactment, all the witnesses who appeared before the Senate Commerce Committee agreed with the need for this legislation, whose purpose was to reduce exposure of the public to all unnecessary hazardous radiation from electronic products by mandating manufacturing standards.[1]

Testimony before the committee specifically confirmed the hazards associated with exposure to radiation. Dr. Philip R. Lee, assistant secretary of the U.S. Department of Health, Education, and Welfare, stated that x-radiation hazards, depending on the dosage, may range from a temporary reddening of the skin all the way to acute damage of the bone marrow. He added that serious delayed chronic effects include leukemia and other cancers, genetic changes, and eye damage.[2]

The subsequent federal laws enacted to control radiation exposure applied only to *new* machines and omitted a most important requirement: to establish the maximum allowable patient exposure per film. Without this requirement, radiation control legislation gives the consumer only a false sense of security.

At the time at which the federal act was passed, hearings held by the Congress concerning the dangers of x-radiation and the need for controls obviously inspired the State of California to start x-ray equipment inspections. Unfortunately, the inspectors have no power to enforce modification of outdated machines.

In the ensuing years, the number of x-ray units registered in California increased constantly, to 39,511 in 1981 from approximately 36,000 in 1978. Over 7,500 x-ray units were inspected in 1981. The total cost for the state's medical and dental radiation control program in that year was $1,426,160.[3]

According to the legislative analyst's 1981 report[3] to the health and welfare committee of the state legislature, the inspections revealed that unsafe conditions were widespread. High-priority machines, i.e., those used continually in hospitals, clinics, and radiologists' offices, were operating with an average of one and a half deficiencies, due to improper adjustment or operation (x-ray beam and film alignment, focal-film distance, film speed and exposure time, etc.). Medium-priority machines, those used intermittently in physicians' and other providers' offices, were operating with an average of two deficiencies of adjustment or operation. The report estimated that ill-health costs from the excess radiation caused by the deficiencies, including medical costs, lost wages, etc., amounted to $3,450 per deficiency per machine.

The report also suggested that the state's radiation control program would raise safety standards by making provision for more frequent inspections of medium- and high-priority machines.

In reality, in the author's opinion, operator competency and safer machines are more significant in maintaining safety standards than frequency of meaningless inspections. High-priority machines are used frequently by trained personnel in hospitals and clinics, and by radiologists. Usually, those institutions use fewer outdated x-ray machines. Independent physicians and other providers, however, are more likely to have less experienced operators and, more often than not, use outdated x-ray machines.

The report blamed existing deficiencies solely on improper adjustment and operation of x-ray machines. It did not address other important deficiencies on older units, such as the absence of equipment which limits the size of the x-ray beam to the affected area only. Therefore, much more body surface may be exposed to radiation than necessary. To cite another problem area: a defective timer which is not backed up by a second timer, as is the case on newer machines, could be especially dangerous, as it might prolong the exposure time needlessly.

Over a period of many years, all California x-ray machines have been inspected two or three times. Yet, they operate now with deficiencies anyway, for the simple reason that inspectors do not have the power to enforce modification of antiquated x-ray equipment; they can only recommend certain improvements but have no jurisdiction to enforce compliance. The fact is that without proper legislation inspections are useless.

To point out the shortcomings of the law, I asked the legislative analyst to answer the following questions pertaining to his report:

1. There are approximately 40,000 registered x-ray units in use in California. How many of those are new units, certified as meeting the federal performance standard for diagnostic x-ray equipment?

2. How many secondhand x-ray units are in use in California?

3. How many x-ray units were ever, by order of inspectors, modified to correct deficiencies?

4. How many x-ray units were ever, by order of inspectors, discarded as unsafe?

Three months later, he answered that he did not have the information I requested.

This answer was not unexpected. Federal and state laws do not regulate outdated x-ray equipment.[4] Therefore, modification or elimination of x-ray units with many deficiencies is not required. For this reason, the information I requested is non-existent.

X-ray machines are operating now in California with an *average* of 1.7 deficiencies. Consequently, some x-ray units could be operating at the higher limit with four or more deficiencies, thus exposing unsuspecting patients to exceptionally high health risks. According to the legislative analyst's report, ill-health cost for each deficiency is estimated by the department of health services to be $3,450 per year. The human cost of serious injuries or genetic mutations caused by x-radiation cannot be estimated in dollar values.

Arthur C. Upton, M.D., director of the National Cancer Institute, reaffirmed the danger of x-radiation before a congressional subcommittee.[5] He testified, in 1978, that exposure could cause injury to body cells and changes in the genes of reproductive cells. Moreover, x-radiation not only may cause increased risk of cancer to the exposed patient but, in the case of a pregnant woman, increased risk of fetal abnormalities.

It follows that deficient x-ray equipment exposing patients to unnecessary high radiation could, indeed, be very dangerous. Therefore, the possibility exists that there is a connection between the deficient x-ray equipment in wide use and the constantly rising cancer incidence and mortality rate.

The most recent 1980 California data show that, according to the bureau of vital statistics, the estimated mortality rate per 100,000 population from cancer has risen from 138.7 in 1965 to 169.0 in 1980. Ironically, it was rising at the same time appropriations for the National Cancer Institute (NCI) increased from $233 million in 1971 to $815 million in 1977, and to over $1 billion in 1980. The increased appropriations for cancer research, unfortunately, have not stopped the trend of a rising cancer mortality rate.

Although the NCI spends $1 billion annually 'fighting cancer," it seems indifferent to the fact that the sale and use of secondhand outdated x-ray equipment, which often exposes patients to high amounts of radiation, is legal and flourishing.

Lung cancer incidence and death rates are constantly rising, but x-rays are not mentioned as a possible cause of lung cancer. In October 1983, a California state health official reported that lung cancer is the leading cause of cancer deaths in California women, and that the lung cancer death rate for California women has doubled since 1970 when the rate was 14 deaths per 100,000 population.[6] Smoking, according to health professionals, is the most significant cause of lung cancer. Yet, smoking by U.S. males declined from 53% to 38% in the last 30 years, and for adult women it declined from 40% to 33%, while the disease rate went up.

About 300 million x-ray examinations are performed annually on the American people and, proportionately, about 40 million on Californians alone. Deficient x-ray equipment is widely used throughout the country, and, combined with sometimes incompetent operators, it poses a considerable danger to the public's health.

A recent *Prevention* magazine article[7] blamed the considerable increase in skin cancer on the sun. It did not mention millions of x-ray examinations in which skin doses vary from a minimum amount to over 80 times as much for the same procedure, depending on the machine used and who is using it. For example, FDA data indicate that chest x-ray dosage varies between one millirem* to over 200 millirems per film. Dental x-ray dosage varies between 40 and over 3,000 millirems per film (see Appendix, page 56). According to the *Prevention* magazine article, records of eight hospitals in Tucson, Arizona, show that the incidence of the worst form of skin cancer, malignant melanoma, jumped 340% over a 10-year period. It is also stated that more people than ever before, and at a much younger age, are afflicted with walking legal

---

*A rem (R), also called roentgen or rad, is a unit of radiation dosage. 1000 millirems (mR), also called milliroentgen or millirads, is equal to one rem. Exposure below five rems (5R), or 5000 mR, is counted as low-level radiation.

blindness (macular degeneration) which, it said, is believed to be directly correlated with exposure to the sun.

If sunshine were a plague, as this article claimed, then our farmers' health should be in jeopardy. There are no statistics to indicate this. The sun shines now as it always has. Our exposure to diagnostic x-radiation is, however, significantly greater now than it has ever been. For protection of the skin from the sun, the article recommended special lotions; for protection of the eyes, sunglasses. Yet, no protection is given to patients' eyes when they undergo head or dental x-ray examination, though x-rays could cause corneal injury and cataracts.

Usually, the news media do not associate increases in cancer incidence with medical radiation. But, according to an article in the *Western Journal of Medicine*[8], the incidence of thyroid cancer increased 300% over the last four decades, and some of this increase may be attributable to radiation-induced tumors caused by radiation treatment of benign conditions, such as acne and ringworm of the scalp. This kind of treatment is no longer practiced today, because of the risk involved.

A *Los Angeles Times* article[9] quoted Dr. Philip Strax, medical director of Gutman Breast Diagnostic Center in New York, as saying, "Twenty years ago, one in 20 women got breast cancer. Today the number is one in 11. It was unusual to find it in women under 40. Now it is not unusual in women under 35. We don't know why." According to the article, Dr. Strax believes all women over 35 should have an annual mammogram (breast x-ray) which he claims gives negligible radiation. Yet, another *Los Angeles Times* article, printed two months later,[10] made the startling disclosure that a study by Dr. Saar Porrath, who has worked in the field of statistics since 1962, revealed that, in the exclusive California suburb of Bel Air, women contract breast cancer at almost three times the rate of poorer women in South Central Los Angeles, and that breast cancer has been shown overwhelmingly to be related to socioeconomic class. The article further states that the causes of breast cancer could be mostly environmental or related to a diet high in meat, such as is consumed by well-to-do Americans.

Such reasoning seems ridiculous. After all, the air quality in residential Bel Air is healthier than that in industrial South Central Los Angeles. And, to my knowledge, there is not a single scientific study which confirms a relationship between a diet high in meat and cancer. There is, however, more than enough evidence that x-radiation could be cancer-causing.

Perhaps, wealthy, well-educated Americans are generally better informed than those who are not so fortunate. (They also are in a better financial position to follow their doctors' advice to undergo routine breast x-ray examinations for cancer detection, at a price of about $100 per examination.) Yet, they are not necessarily well-informed about the dangers associated with radiation exposure and the fact that studies have shown that the female breast is particularly radiosensitive. X-ray examinations, especially those in which deficient x-ray equipment is used, could be instrumental in the future development of breast and other cancers.

The fact is that twenty years ago when mammography was scarcely used, *one woman in twenty* developed breast cancer. Now, when mammography is performed on more than 2 million women annually, the number is *one in eleven*, and cancer of the breast has become a very serious medical problem for women. The relation between the higher cancer incidence and mammography has not been investigated.

According to the report of a delegation that visited the People's Republic of China in 1977,[11] mammography for breast examinations was not used in China. It may be significant that the incidence of breast cancer for Shanghai women in 1975 was 15.16 in 100,000, as compared with 64.4 in 100,000 U.S. white females in 1969-71. According to the *Los Angeles Times* article, the current Bel Air rate per 100,000 white women is an astonishing 142.

It appears from the published record that health professionals are not concerned with the dangers and consequences of diagnostic x-rays, in spite of the fact that these dangers have been documented over the years and should be well known.

In 1903, Nobel Prize winner Pierre Curie, in his acceptance speech, warned the world for the first time about the great dangers of radiation. Little did he know then that both his wife, Marie, a well-known pioneer in the discovery of radium, and his daughter, Irene, would die from radiation-induced sickness — leukemia.

Another pioneer, Dr. Edmund Kells of New Orleans, who introduced dental radiography in the United States, himself fell victim to radiation as many others in this field did.

Some dentists have suffered from cancer of the hand caused by holding x-ray film in the mouths of patients. They have solved the problem for themselves by letting the patients hold the film or clamp it in their teeth.

Then there are the Hiroshima survivors; Utah residents who in disproportionate numbers died from cancer after nuclear weapon tests fallout; nuclear submarine workers who develop higher than normal percentages of leukemia, and many other victims of radiation. To name one, Adelle Davis, a well-known nutritionalist, developed bone cancer and died two years after extensive x-ray examinations requested by her insurance carrier. Like many other radiation victims, she knew what caused her cancer and tried to tell the public of the danger. But outcries such as hers have fallen, and will continue to fall, on deaf ears as long as the medical establishment claims otherwise.

In 1979, a White House task force, acknowledging the fact that radiation is cumulative and could be carcinogenic, called for reducing the exposure of Americans to man-made radiation, particularly medical x-rays. It urged doctors to be cautious in ordering x-rays and encouraged patients to avoid unnecessary x-ray examinations. Yet, this task force overlooked the fact that federal and state laws permit the use of outdated, secondhand x-ray equipment, which sometimes exposes patients to high levels of radiation. Without elimination of antiquated x-ray equipment, an effective reduction of exposure to man-made radiation is impossible.

The National Cancer Institute stated in 1978 that x-rays could be cancer-causing.[5] Yet, this institute did not sponsor any measures to prevent patient overexposure to radiation.

The NCI statement referred to a study sponsored by the U.S. Food and Drug Administration (FDA), and being continued by the NCI, which reaffirms the fact that frequently repeated relatively low radiation doses pose some future risk of breast cancer, primarily, and that the risk may be cumulative.

In general, the statement said, cancer occurs in greater numbers in certain organs more frequently than others after irradiation. The organs affected, in decreasing order, are the female breast, thyroid gland, blood-forming organs, lung, gastro-intestinal tract, and skeleton.

In spite of the dangers of x-radiation, the tide of x-ray use is constantly rising in the United States, as shown by the FDA statement to Congress in 1978.[12]

The agency conducted two national surveys of x-ray use that showed examinations increased 24 percent between 1964 and 1970. At that rate, it estimated, x-ray examinations would reach 241 million annually by 1977 and, by extrapolation, about 300 million in 1983.

With the introduction in 1973 of the computerized tomography (CT) scanner, the number of x-ray examinations further increased, along with the average radiation exposure per examination. The agency said approximately 700 CT scanners were in use for 2 million patients a year.

The report also stated that mammography (in which relatively large amounts of radiation are delivered to a particularly radiosensitive tissue) was scarcely used as recently as 15 years ago and, by 1978, was performed on approximately 2 million women in the United States annually.

Of the 270,000 dental and medical machines in use, the testimony pointed out, only 19% were x-ray systems manufactured and sold after August 1, 1974, therefore meeting the FDA's new performance standards. In addition, only 80,000 machine operators were licensed or certified out of an estimated 110,000 to 170,000 people who operate medical x-ray equipment.

Yet, the FDA had no programs for correcting those significant deficiencies. As is evident from this 1978 statement, 81% of all x-ray units in use at the time were substandard; also, from 30,000 to 90,000 operators of x-ray equipment were not certified or licensed.

Instead of working toward the elimination of substandard x-ray equipment and toward mandatory training of operators, the agency started to conduct two *voluntary* programs designed to reduce x-ray exposure. One is known as DENT, or Dental Exposure Normalization Technique, and the other is a mammography program known as BENT, or Breast Exposure: Nationwide Trends. The radiation control agency sends x-ray exposure cards to dental and medical facilities. There they are exposed and then returned for analysis. Facilities that show excessive exposure are then visited to demonstrate the changes needed to produce better quality radiographs with minimum patient exposure. The rest is left to the good intentions of the equipment owner. These programs are useless as long as there is no maximum allowable exposure per film established, operators of x-ray equipment are not properly trained and licensed, and outdated x-ray equipment is not required to be modified, upgraded, or discarded.

While operators of automobiles are tested for their driving capability and must obtain driver's licenses, many states have allowed untested or poorly trained individuals to operate the potentially lethal x-ray machine.[13] On August 13, 1981, Congress finally enacted legislation calling for federal standards for accrediting training programs and licensing or credentialing individuals who operate radiographic equipment, *exempting* dentists, physicians, and chiropractors. The states are expected to fully comply with this legislation within a specified three-year period.

In light of the above, it is not surprising that, according to government surveys, more than one-third of dental x-ray machines, and almost one-half of breast x-ray machines, emitted *unacceptable* levels of radiation.[13] It appears that the Food and Drug Administration does not make a practice of informing the consumer about existing dose variations and possible risks involved in undergoing x-ray examination. Their publications for consumer information minimize those risks. For example, "Get the Picture on . . . Dental X-Rays,"[14] states that "less is known about the effects from *small* amounts of radiation, such as used in dental x-rays." (Emphasis added.)

The fact is, as Dr. Loren F. Mills, of the FDA, stated in a December 1979 letter to the *Journal of the American Dental Association*, dental radiography requires relatively high exposure and dose rates, and the critical areas involved in dental radiography are likely to be the red bone marrow of the jaw, the thyroid gland, and the lens of the eye.

The thyroid gland is second in radiation sensitivity after the female breast. Dentists seem to be ignorant of this fact and, when taking x-rays, seldom use special collars for thyroid gland protection. According to the *Western Journal of Medicine*, November 1979, *the incidence of thyroid cancer has increased 300% over the last four decades.*

It must be assumed that irradiation of the brain in dental radiography is also unavoidable. This additional danger was not mentioned by Dr. Mills but explained by John W. Gofman, M.D., in his recently published book, *Radiation and Human Health*, in which he associates brain irradiation from dental x-rays with an increased risk of brain cancer, especially in children.

A Department of Health, Education, and Welfare 1979 publication[15] stated that no one knows exactly what causes breast cancer; so there is nothing anyone can do to prevent the disease. Should breast cancer develop, it assured, the chances of obtaining "effective treatment and coping with the disease are improved." It also cited a National Cancer Institute recommendation of mammography for cancer detection in women aged 50 and over but, nevertheless, cautioned that women should ask how much radiation each breast will receive. A maximum of 1,000 millirems (mR) per breast was advised.

This 1979 pamphlet indicated that about one woman in fourteen will develop the disease sometime during her lifetime. By 1983, the number had risen to one in eleven.

In spite of the previously mentioned FDA-sponsored study[5] reaffirming the cumulative danger of relatively low radiation doses, the 1979 pamphlet maintains that no one knows exactly what causes breast cancer; however, without stating that radiation is cancer-inducing, it implies it by advising women to avoid exposures over 1,000 mR per breast. It is not explained how this could be achieved. If radiation were not carcinogenic, then the dosage would be of no consequence. But, if radiation is, in fact, cancer-causing, then the question must be asked why no further protective steps were taken after 1978 FDA data showed that 81% of the x-ray units used were substandard, and at least 30,000 unlicensed, untrained operators were performing x-ray examinations. As stated before, nearly one-half of breast x-ray machines emitted unacceptable levels of radiation, too.[13]

An article in *Consumer Reports*[16] goes even further by simply stating that women who require mammography tests should insist on a dose of less than 1,000 mR per breast.

It appears from this statement that the writer is comparing x-ray equipment to something like a spigot whose flow is easily controllable. The amount of x-ray exposure, in fact, depends on several factors beyond control in an outdated machine, among which are the capacity of the machine to limit the beam to the area of concern and precise limitation of exposure to the least time required.

Between 1979 and 1983, several prominent physicians reassured the public that mammography is the most effective tool in detecting breast cancer, and that the risks involved are very small. One physician claimed that mammography exposure involves no risk if modern equipment is used. Another one gave the amount of radiation exposure for this examination as precisely 2,000 mR, and others stated that exposure varied between low and extremely low. The fact is that no maximum allowable exposure limits have been established, and doses vary dramatically from low to high between different facilities. Therefore, stating that breast x-ray examination exposure is of a specific amount, or that it varies between low and extremely low, is not factual but misleading.

Dr. Wende Logan, a radiologist, appearing on the Phil Donahue TV show,[17] recommended yearly mammography for women over 50, and claimed that since 1975 mammography exposure has been reduced and picture quality has been improved twenty times. With all these alleged improvements, why then did she also advise women to ask of their physicians how much radiation they will receive, and why did she also caution them to make sure that "special equipment" is used in those examinations. Her "recommended dose" was a maximum of 500 mR per film. She did not, however, propose a practical method for the woman patient to ascertain that this level of radiation will, in fact, be administered and that proper equipment will be used.

In response to my inquiry concerning the safety of their x-ray equipment, a well-known Los Angeles medical facility stated that all diagnostic radiographic equipment located in their department of radiologic sciences meets or exceeds the requirements as outlined by the federal performance standard.[18]

The FDA computer printout of certified x-ray equipment used by facilities in Los Angeles, however, shows that, after the new standard went into effect, the Los Angeles medical facility in question acquired only 21 certified x-ray units. To my knowledge, the facility uses a total of 54 x-ray units. Therefore, if I am correct, 33 x-ray units are *not* federally certified, while the facility claims that *all* of its units meet or exceed the federal standard. To my subsequent inquiries concerning this discrepancy, I received no reply.

I requested information about their dose rate from a medical facility that suggested breast x-ray to my wife while they assured her that mammography radiation exposure was very small. At the same time, I asked local and state radiation control agencies for information pertaining to this facility's mammographic unit. I received three conflicting letters in response to my requests. The medical facility in question informed me that its dose rate is 140 mR per film to the mid-breast. The county's radiation management agency stated that a mammography exam at that facility delivers about 150 mR to the breast (a minimum of two films is required per breast), and the state's radiation control unit informed me that the cranio-caudal (mid-breast) exposure in 1977 was measured at 500 mR. The fact that I received three different answers to my question confirms my suspicion that it is almost impossible to obtain accurate information concerning x-ray examinations, unless x-ray equipment testing is performed by an independent agency.

As mentioned earlier, radiologist Dr. Wende Logan claimed in 1983 that, since 1975, mammography exposure has been reduced and the picture quality has been improved, 20 times. The credibility of such assertions is put in doubt by the U.S. comptroller general's report dated December 1979.[13] This report states that 45 states had surveyed 3,253 of about 4,000 x-ray units used for mammography in the United States, resulting in identification of 1,496, or 46%, of the surveyed units, with either excessively high or unusually low exposure. (The latter, being of poor diagnostic quality, may require additional pictures to be taken, without certainty of improving the picture quality, but with the possibility of further exposing the patient needlessly to harmful radiation.) According to information received in 1981 from the Department of Health and Human Services, Bureau of Radiological Health, only 727 mammographic units nationwide, or about 18% of all units in use (4,000), had been certified at that time as meeting the FDA's performance standard for diagnostic x-ray equipment. (See Appendix, page 57.)

If 46% of the units surveyed in 1979 showed excessively high or unusually low exposure, and only 18% of the total number in use in 1981 had met government standards, are we to believe Dr. Logan's assurances two years later?

A good example of how high some exposures could be is given in an article by the Minnesota Department of Health,[19] published in 1977, in which the department contended that in Minnesota the highest exposure found in mammography machines was 5,000 mR, and it added that startling statement, "In round numbers, for a typical exam with two views, a woman received about 21,000 mR." The article went on to say that, eventually, after working with the facility in question, the department had managed to reduce exposure by 13,000 mR per examination, obtaining acceptable mammograms by using 2,000 mR for one view. This resulted in approximately 8,000 mR per exam. While the health department's effort may be commendable, this is still four times more than the recommended dosage, which is a maximum of 1,000 mR per breast. One film should deliver no more than 500 mR, Dr. Logan says; a minimum of two films is needed for one breast examination.

The *voluntary* program known as "Breast Exposure: Nationwide Trends (BENT) is being implemented by state radiation control agencies on a nationwide basis. As of January 1978, 19 states had received data showing that the average exposure was 920 mR for a single film,[20] which means that the average (one breast only) examination, requiring at least two films, could have been 1,840 mR, or 840 mR more than the recommended dosage of a maximum of 1,000 mR per one breast. A complete mammography examination (involving two breasts) requires at least four films. Based on an average exposure of 920 mR per film and considering wide dose variations, the single maximum exposure could be ten times as much, and this would be extremely dangerous to a woman.

Such is the case in California where, in 1979, the maximum breast x-ray exposure was recorded at 10,700 mR per film, 20 times higher than Dr. Logan recommended.[21] Official 1981 California data indicate that x-ray machines are operating with an average of 1.7 deficiencies.[3] Therefore, some machines could operate with four and more deficiencies and endanger women considerably.

The X-Ray Information Book, by Priscilla W. Laws, Ph.D., and Ralph Nader's Public Citizen Health Research Group,[22] appears to be a do-it-yourself guide for the consumer on how to minimize exposure to x-rays. Instead of examining the causes of unnecessary radiation overexposure and proposing remedial actions, the authors make ludicrous suggestions as to how the consumer may minimize the exposure to x-rays by learning to evaluate his physician, dentist, radiologist, and x-ray technologist, as well as their facilities, and by assessing some of the more obvious procedures employed by the people who operate the x-ray equipment (p. 63 of the book). This advice would seem to be somewhat disingenous, particularly as it was extended to severely ill or hospitalized patients.

In his foreword to the book, Dr. Sidney M. Wolfe, Director of the research group, warns that there is an extensive and constantly increasing use of x-rays in the United States. He refers to an estimate published by *Medical Economics*[23] that 30% of diagnostic x-ray procedures are unnecessary and claims that at least half the diagnostic x-ray examination doses are unnecessary and could be detrimental to the health of the American people.

This book seems to say that the situation is dangerous, but that the responsibility for correcting it rests with the patient and not with the professionals who perform x-ray examinations. This is surely preposterous. Some health professionals are quite ignorant concerning x-radiation doses, x-ray equipment quality, and the dangers associated with those examinations. The public has a right to expect that those who perform the examinations are properly trained and possess credentials that certify their competence as equipment operators, also, that they use federally certified x-ray machines.

Radiation control agencies seem helpless to improve the effectiveness of the control laws. Professional organizations such as the American Academy of Dental Radiology, and others*, whose concern should be the health of the patients they serve, are silent on the subject. Even investigative reporters do not question the unregulated use of often unsafe x-ray equipment for diagnostic purposes.

To appease public concern for radiation safety, the control laws were enacted. The responsibility for protecting the consumer against unnecessary radiation exposure was given to the FDA's

---

*The American Association of Physicists in Medicine, American Dental Association, American Medical Association, American Society of Radiologic Technologists, Health Physics Society, and Ralph Nader's Public Citizen Health Research Group.

bureau of radiological health which was instrumental in enactment of the laws.

This legislation was an important first step, but any further meaningful regulatory legislation has been stopped by the medical and dental establishments. They object strongly to any federal or state interference in their practices. Through strong lobbying efforts and substantial campaign contributions to legislators, they have succeeded in killing attempts at further regulation.

The absurdity of the present law is evident from the fact that no maximum allowable patient exposure per film has been established. Without limiting exposures, it should be evident, the control of radiation is impossible.

The cost to the public of unregulated x-ray overexposure is enormous; arguably as much as $792 million annually. The state of California estimates that excess radiation received by patients over a one-year period due to deficiencies in adjustment or operation of machines results in ill-health costs of $3,450 for each deficiency. Since x-ray units in medical facilities in the state are operating with an average of 1.7 deficiencies per unit, and there are approximately 21,000 medical units in use, the ill-health cost from radiation overexposure is over $123 million in California alone, each year. The annual cost for the nation can be estimated at over $790 million.

II.

DENTAL X-RAY DANGERS

Informed consumers today are aware of the necessity to protect themselves. The days are gone when patients accepted medical and dental procedures without question. The problem is that questions of dental x-ray safety are turned aside by professionals with assurances that there is no danger, or at the very worst, that there is an acceptable minimum. The truth is that many dentists, among others, are inadequately educated in the safe use of x-rays.

Dental x-rays are much more dangerous than we are told. The consumer who undergoes dental radiography is not informed about the exposure doses, the danger of radiation, or the vulnerability of organs of the head and neck region which are also irradiated during the process.

Few consumers take the initiative to ask a dentist if the x-ray equipment is up-to-date and certified as meeting the federal performance standard; or ask if it is a secondhand, substandard machine. Eighty-one percent of the machines in use in 1978 were built before standards were set. There were no controls over their performance then, and there are still no controls today. Substandard machines are lacking important safety features which help reduce patient exposure, such as lead-lined, open-end cones to reduce scatter radiation; electronic timers to shorten exposure time to a fraction of a second; film-holding devices for better positioning; and proper filtration to remove harmful but not useful low energy x-rays from the beam.

Six years ago, when I started this investigation, my perception regarding dental x-rays was similar to that expressed in the California legislative analyst's report.[3] According to this report, ill-health costs from improper use of dental x-ray machines are significantly lower (10 to 12 times) than ill-health costs from either medium- or high-priority medical x-ray machines. This view, that dental x-ray dangers are minimal, was substantiated by occasional articles appearing in the news media.

Yet, every day of my investigation brought to light new and startling surprises concerning wide variations in dental x-ray doses. One facility, for example, could expose the patient to 40 millirems per film, while, at another facility, for the same procedure, a patient could be exposed to 4,000 mR, as California Department of Health Services data indicate (see Appendix, page 58). At the same time, this high dose was irradiating the brain, eyes, thyroid gland, and bone marrow in the jaw.

Consequently, I read books on radiology and wrote hundreds of letters in an attempt to confirm the reliability of my findings. Not all my letters were answered. The replies I did receive were mostly evasive and sometimes far from the truth.

In its publication, *Radiation Protection in Dental Practice*,[24] the Board of Dental Examiners cautioned dentists about the risks involved in overexposure and about their professional obligations. It is important, the book stressed, to keep radiation exposure "as low as possible consistent with diagnostic requirements." Dentists were reminded that they control half the x-ray machines in use today and, therefore, have a professional obligation to "eliminate unnecessary radiation" from their practices.

The fact is that the elimination of unnecessary radiation in dental practice is unattainable as long as there are no set standards for *all* x-ray equipment. The federal performance standard covers only new equipment manufactured after 1974. It is important to stress that all x-ray machines manufactured prior to that are exempt from meeting any standards. (See **Appendix,** page 59.)

Radiology specialists within the dental profession are aware of the danger, and some have supported legislation raising the standards.

For instance, Dr. A. B. Reiskin, a radiology professor at the University of Connecticut, in testimony before a congressional subcommittee in 1978,[25] opined that dentists are inadequately educated in the use of x-rays or their adverse effects. He suggested that a significant number of routine diagnostic x-rays were unnecessary and of a higher dosage than required by newer technology. Overexposure and overutilization occur, he said, because of inadequate education and the lack of meaningful guidelines and controls.

Dr. Reiskin recommended minimum educational requirements for the prescriber of x-ray examinations as well as the machine operators. Additionally, he urged quality assurance programs in dental offices and precise recordkeeping, including estimated exposures. He underscored the importance of periodic inspection and calibration of machines, x-ray beam-guiding and -restricting devices, and continuing education requirements for all practicing dentists.

None of these recommendations were enacted into law.

III.

FOOD AND DRUG
ADMINISTRATION'S
OPPOSITE POINT OF VIEW

The Food and Drug Administration commissioner, Dr. Donald Kennedy, in his statement to Congress,[12] during the congressional subcommittee hearings in 1978, ignored the recommendations made by Dr. A. B. Reiskin of the University of Connecticut.[25] Dr. Kennedy recommended, instead, that remedial measures be taken on a voluntary basis. In his testimony, he revealed the startling statistics mentioned in Chapter I (page 13): only 19% of x-ray machines in use were meeting the government standard effective since 1974; only about 50% of the operators were certified or licensed to use x-ray equipment; and the use of x-ray examinations had increased 24% in the six years the FDA had been conducting surveys before funds ran out.

Nevertheless, according to the commissioner, the FDA's programs consisted essentially of establishing toothless recommendations for good radiation practices and of educating health personnel as well as consumers. He did not refer to the fact that neither recommendations nor education will build into older x-ray machines the needed safety features to keep to a minimum the amount of radiation. Such safety features are required for x-ray equipment manufactured after 1974 and are described in *A Practitioner's Guide to the Diagnostic X-Ray Equipment Standard.*[4]

The commissioner supported recommendations for improving user practices voluntarily, rather than strict requirements, because, he said, the issues were complex and "good practices tend to evolve over time." At the time, the FDA had some recommendations in effect, and he assured the legislators it was developing other safety guides. They were to be used, presumably, when and if practitioners felt like using them. He did, however, express concern that scientific studies, partly funded by the FDA, showed an association between x-ray exposure and leukemia, and other cancers, in children but argued that the most effective equipment regulation would not guarantee minimal exposure any more than "automobile standards assure safety in driving." The commissioner's reasoning in comparing safety in driving to x-ray equipment regulation is ridiculous. Only effective regulation of *all* equipment through strictly enforced performance standards will reduce patient overexposure, just as only effective regulation of auto pollution control devices will improve air quality.

If the FDA expects to improve dangerous equipment performance with recommendations only, then it should also be possible to control air pollution by simply making recommendations. The best education will not protect us against unregulated air-pollution machinery, nor will it protect us against overexposure by unregulated older x-ray equipment.

As a result of the FDA's "logic" (not opposed by the medical establishment), which is impossible to explain rationally, the federal performance standard does not apply to antiquated x-ray machines still in use, and does not require them to be modified, upgraded, or discarded. (See Appendix, page 59.)

When John Villforth, director of the FDA's bureau of radiological health, testified five years earlier before a Senate committee (see Appendix, page 60), he stressed the importance of the bureau's performance standard for new diagnostic x-ray equipment as "by far the most complex and far-reaching in its impact on the public's health." The significance, he said, was that 90% of exposure to man-made radiation came from diagnostic x-radiation.

By 1982, Villforth had switched from stressing the importance of built-in performance standards to emphasizing operator expertise. He replied to my complaint concerning unmodified older units widely used in dental and medical offices that these machines were efficient when "properly maintained and utilized." (See Appendix, page 63.) The bureau's experience, he indicated, showed that equipment age is far less important than training, supervision, and the practices of the operators.

Dr. James W. Miller, also of the bureau of radiological health, expressed this same point of view in his reply to my 1978 letter to the FDA about high dental x-ray exposure levels and free trade of unregulated used equipment. "This equipment," he said, "is not considered to be a major factor" in overexposure, because manufacturers started meeting proposed federal standards several years before they took effect (see Appendix, page 66). The problem in dentistry, he added, is the manner in which personnel use the equipment, a difficult area to regulate and one over which the FDA has no authority. (See Appendix, page 68.) The FDA seems to be in a dilemma. On the one hand, it stresses the importance of training and good personnel practices and, on the other, admits its impotence to achieve them.

I believe overexposures are rampant throughout the country. If an old x-ray machine has no built-in safety features, such as a proper x-ray beam restriction device, this could only be corrected through modification of the equipment, and not through proper maintenance or excellent operating practices, as the federal regulators contend. The same applies to similar safety features. Overexposures from these units are blamed, nevertheless, not on outmoded equipment but generally on the lack of proper training, supervision, and skills of the personnel operating old machines.

IV.

CALIFORNIA RADIATION CONTROL REGULATIONS

As it stands now, the law does not protect consumers from the hazard of overradiation from outmoded x-ray machines or incompetent operators. Protective legislation will not be passed until consumers demand that their rights to health be placed above the rights of the medical and dental establishments to remain unregulated.

California radiation control regulations[26] follow the federal example in not providing adequate protection for the consumer. State regulations protect not the patient but only the user of x-ray machines, who needs demonstrate to the Health Department's satisfaction only achievement of "equivalent protection" through means other than modification of equipment. (See Appendix, page 70.)

It is impossible to improve patient protection, however, without equipment modification. California regulations, like their federal counterparts, do not require it. As is stated in the law, users' radiation protection could be achieved through other means than modification, such as operating x-ray equipment from behind a leaded shield. Consumer protection is left to the consumer.

According to the FDA commissioner's 1978 report, only 19% of x-ray units were certified as meeting the federal standard. This means that 81% of all x-ray equipment in use was not certified. These machines may be lacking even today in important safety features; yet, they are not required to be changed or discarded. (See Appendix, page 59.)

It took five years to discover where and how to obtain a list of dental offices that use modern x-ray equipment. The source is the FDA. In 1977, though, when I first started inquiring, the California bureau of radiological health replied that it did not keep records that would provide that information and made no reference to the agency that does. (See Appendix, page 71).

During the past 14 years, my family has been treated in four different dental facilities, and not a single one of them used modern x-ray machines, equipped with open-end cones, electronic timers, thyroid-protective collars, or film-holding devices. Even so, all four of them were eager to take x-rays, one of them even being so bold as to refuse routine examination of the patient before taking x-rays. Upon my complaint, the unprofessional behavior was justified in a letter to me stating, "Our technicians and facilities meet all California standards for safety and competence . . . ." (See Appendix, page 72.)

Unfortunately, nothing could have been further from the truth. I found that in 1976 the x-ray equipment of the dental facility in question was "inspected," and the results of this "inspection" indicated exposures ranging from 619 to 1,735 millirems per film (see Appendix, page 72), as compared with exposures from up-to-date equipment which range from 100 to 300 mR per film. The exposure at this facility was about six times more than needed for good radiographs.

I received no satisfactory answers to my many complaints to the state agencies concerning this particular dentist who uses outdated x-ray equipment, overexposes patients, and insists on first taking x-rays before giving an oral examination. According to the California radiation control agency's own explanation, dentists are specifically exempt from the bureau's jurisdiction, and the bureau's program "deals only with the registration and inspection of dental x-ray equipment." (See Appendix, page 71.) Yet, no one seems to be questioning the absurdity of this activity.

If the California department of health would suddenly declare that Los Angeles restaurants were exempt from their jurisdiction, but that, nevertheless, the law requires them to inspect those restaurants periodically, the law would be laughed at. Such logic would simply be unacceptable. The state's procedures would be declared incompetent as wasting taxpayers' money on useless inspections. So-called inspections of x-ray equipment have been conducted in California since 1968, and yet not a single law has been enacted to make them effective.

In answer to my complaint in 1978 that antiquated x-ray machines are widely used in Los Angeles County dental offices and are a hazard to patients, the director of the health services department wrote that for over ten years the county has contracted with the state for periodic inspections of all dental facilities, many of which have been checked several times. In addition, he wrote, incidents and "other concerns" have been investigated and citations issued where appropriate. (See Appendix, page 73.) Nowhere did he say that California regulations require only incidents involving x-ray *users* to be reported. Moreover, those dental facilities contained equipment at that time, 81% of which was *exempt from any regulations*.

Much like the county health department, the state health department restated in a 1979 letter: "The department is responsible for inspecting dental (and many other) x-ray machines to protect against unsafe levels of radiation . . . and does have the legal right to cite violations and to require correction of hazardous conditions involving x-ray machines." (See Appendix, page 75.)

These claims are contradicted by California Radiation Control Regulations, Title 17, Health, Sections 30252 and 30297, according to which patient overexposures to radiation are not required to be reported. (See Appendix, page 70.)

The disparity between the Department's professed concern for public safety and the harsh reality of California law which makes no substantial provision for the protection of the public in the area of x-radiation must be attributed either to ignorance of the law or to a deliberate effort by the Department of Health to calm public apprehension with misinformation.

One month after the state health department's assurance of protection against overexposure, the supervisor of the state x-radiation control unit contradicted this, saying that the state, indeed, does not have regulations "covering many factors which closely affect patient exposure." The supervisor referred to the current practice of making *recommendations* to dentists for correction. The futility of such recommendations is underscored by his statement that cases of excessive radiation were "obviously where our recommendations were not followed." He added that state regulations were nearly always copied from federal ones for uniformity. They are copied, it seems, whether or not they do the job. (See Appendix, page 77.)

Apparently, uniformity is the goal, and not concern about antiquated x-ray equipment. The majority of dental offices have units which lack important safety features such as open-end lead-lined cones to restrict the beam, electronic timers, thyroid-protective collars, film-holding and cone-positioning devices — all features that reduce patient exposure. The state control unit, in reality, does not *control* overexposures but only records them. Even though inspectors are fully aware of the fact that many dental offices use machines which overexpose patients to radiation, the law does not require corrective measures to be taken, nor has the public been made aware of this serious health hazard.

Identification and control of hazardous x-ray equipment is impossible because the American Dental Association opposes legislation requiring the setting of performance standards for all x-ray equipment, old as well as new. Without appropriate legislation, inspections are meaningless. They are comparable to building inspections without established building safety standards.

Considering all the facts, it is not surprising that, after eleven years of periodical dental x-ray equipment "inspections" in California, in 1979 exposures were still ranging widely from 45 to 4,106 mR per film (see Appendix, page 58), whereas modern dental x-ray equipment exposure ranges are from 100 to 300 mR per film. According to a federal publication,[27] acceptable dental x-ray exposure for quality radiographs may vary from 100 to 500 mR per film. In my opinion, such a wide dose variation should not be acceptable to anyone, least of all the consumer. The publication in question also states that dental x-ray examinations have shown exposures at skin level ranging from 100 mR to 50 times as much for each film, depending on the facility. (See Appendix, page 78.)

Though I had lengthy correspondence with radiation control agencies, they all neglected to point out that many dental and medical facilities use older, secondhand x-ray units that are not certified, although x-ray equipment manufactured after 1974 may be assumed to be certified as meeting the federal performance standard. I came across this information only through considerable research of this subject. When I started inquiries regarding the prevalence of certified x-ray machines in Los Angeles, the state health department informed me that purchasers of old or new x-ray machines were not required to notify the county of the equipment's certification, or lack of it. Also, the department had no information about the location of certified machines. In 1982, the county of Los Angeles health department claimed that as much as 20% of all machines in use in the county were certified as meeting the federal standard, but was unable to provide a breakdown of the certified units by location. (See Appendix, page 79.)

Through further inquiries, I discovered that, of four dental offices located in my vicinity and using a total of 10 x-ray machines, only one had a machine that was certified as meeting the standard. One wonders how representative that is of other neighborhood dental offices.

In May 1982, a Los Angeles TV station presented a series on x-ray dangers.[28] During the series, which placed the same misguided emphasis on inspections without enforcement, the reporter concluded that not enough inspections are performed; that some x-ray units "have not been looked at for 15 years," and that, therefore, patient overexposures occur. An improved inspection service, however, is now supposed to correct everything within five years, viewers were assured. Nevertheless, the county department of health services claimed in 1978 that all x-ray facilities are periodically inspected to ensure compliance with legal standards. "This activity has been carried out . . . for over ten years . . . and *many units have been checked several times* (emphasis added)." (See Appendix, page 73.)

Over a period of many years, however, although many units were inspected several times, there has been little effect on patient radiation exposure. The simple reason is that inspectors cannot enforce modification of pre-1974 x-ray equipment, they can only recommend certain improvements, and a large percentage of the units in use are pre-1974. Therefore, as long as federal and state laws exempt these machines from any regulations, and in many instances they emit excessive radiation, the inspections serve no practical purpose.

During the 1982 TV program, the California state x-ray regulator stated, "Perhaps one of the weaknesses we have is that there is no real penalty if a user fails to abide by the law — it is a misdemeanor." This statement confounded me. To my knowledge, there is not a single federal or state law enacted which would, in any way, regulate medical or dental practice.

Therefore, within a week, I wrote asking him to clarify his public statement. Specifically, I asked for a written statement that it is a misdemeanor to buy second-hand equipment and, in using it, expose patients to excessive radiation. I inquired about the specific section of the law under which users could be legally cited or fined; the number of units in use in California; the number meeting federal standards; and their location. To date, I have not received a reply to these questions.

V.

THE AMERICAN DENTAL ASSOCIATION'S VIEW

The American Dental Association (ADA) misinforms the public because it wants to avoid any government regulation of dental x-rays. It has worked for years to defeat proposed legislation with much success. The public, meanwhile, has minimal protection from excessive radiation exposure or from old, unsafe x-ray machines.

In a special issue of the *Journal of the American Dental Association* (JADA), entitled "A Consumer's Guide to Dental Health, 1982," certain assertions were put forward that have yet to be substantiated. The guide claimed that federal and state agencies try to ensure that dental x-ray equipment is working properly, that state agencies inspect equipment regardless of manufacturing date, and that existing regulations provide a sound measure of protection. In light of widely used outdated x-ray equipment, and dramatic dose variations, which could range from 40 to over 3,000 millirems per film, such claims have no factual foundation.

In 1977, a JADA article[29] gave a detailed explanation of federal regulations, stating that the federal performance standard, which became effective three years earlier, is primarily directed toward the manufacturer, and *most practicing dentists need not be knowledgeable about the details of the standard* (emphasis added).

JADA's consumer guide points out that the federal standard requires several safety features to be built into new machines so that patients receive minimum radiation, but makes no mention of the fact that in 1982 only about 20% of all dental x-ray equipment in use was certified as meeting this standard. Furthermore, the ADA's lobbying efforts prevented government endeavors to standardize all x-ray equipment. The association's success in defeating government efforts is best illustrated by the JADA 1981 article entitled "Self-Regulation vs. Government Intervention."[30]

According to the article, as of September 1980, the ADA had testified three times during the preceding 14 months *in opposition* to proposals imposing federal standards and reorganizing administrative responsibilities.

In the past 15 years, the U.S. Congress and the executive branch have studied a number of proposals designed to alleviate concerns about radiation and its potential hazards. The JADA 1981 article refers to a number of bills that were introduced concerning radiation safety, including some[31] which were to direct the government to set radiation standards for, and conduct regular inspections of, diagnostic and other x-ray systems. *Those bills were defeated.*

In 1981, the Congress approved, in the absence of ADA opposition, legislation calling for federal standards for accrediting training programs and licensing or credentialing individuals who operate radiographic equipment, *excluding dentists, physicians, and chiropractors.*

The principle that it is all right to regulate people but wrong to regulate existing machines seems to be firmly established. As for monitoring potentially dangerous older x-ray units, Congressman Henry A. Waxman wrote me concerning the above-mentioned bill, that, at the time it was discussed, his subcommittee and the Senate committee involved also discussed the difficulty of finding and regulating older x-ray machines that might have had several owners, and decided problems could be best reduced by correctly training personnel in their use.

I disagree with the legislators' conclusion. Our radiation control agencies, which are well aware that many units overexpose patients, would be able to control older x-ray machines, even if they had had several owners and were difficult to trace, if appropriate legislation were enacted.

According to JADA's 1981 article, significant improvements have been made to reduce radiation with x-ray equipment manufactured under the new standards. They include the use of filtration, beam-direction devices, open-end cones, electronic timers, lead aprons and thyroid-protective collars, and film-holding and cone-positioning devices. The fact is that only a small percentage of patients benefit, since modern dental x-ray machines manufactured under the new standards are scarce and difficult to locate. Our legislators and the FDA make a dangerous assumption that, with properly trained personnel, antiquated x-ray equipment will perform satisfactorily.

At last in 1982, after considerable endeavor, I received the FDA computer printout of Los Angeles County dental and medical facilities that, since 1974, had installed new certified x-ray units. It was obvious to me that only one unit was certified out of 10 in my vicinity. Unfortunately, the dentist who uses that unit, equipped with a safer open-end cone, also uses two uncertified units. They are equipped with pointed plastic cones, which are a major source of secondary radiation. Incidentally, the ADA does not recommend them. In addition, not a single dentist known to my family uses thyroid-protective collars or film-holding and cone-positioning devices. Nevertheless, JADA's consumer's guide to dental health states that less is known about the effects from *small* amounts of radiation, such as that used in dental x-rays. The ADA appears willing to accept the risks to patients from something it knows little about.

It is important to stress, once again, that secondhand x-ray equipment, which sometimes overexposes patients, is not required to be improved or scrapped. This older equipment is widely used throughout the country, in spite of the reality that any exposure to radiation involves some risk, the degree of which increases as the amount of radiation increases. The effects of radiation are, after all, cumulative.

In 1979, thirty-eight states surveyed over 35,000 dental x-ray units. Analysis indicated that exposures from 36% of them appeared excessively high. (See Appendix, page 60.)

The FDA published data in 1981 from 1,036 of their dental equipment surveys showing maximum/minimum exposures. They varied between 41 mR and 83 times as much per film for the same procedure. Also, the size of surface exposure varied considerably (see Appendix, page 56). The fact that one unit of the 1,036 surveyed had the highest radiation of 3,418 mR per film suggests that as many as 145 machines of the estimated 150,000 dental x-ray units in use in this country might be likewise jeopardizing patients.

As shown in the surveys, dental x-ray exposures vary widely. It is time a maximum limit for patient exposure per film is established, and also a requirement to discard antiquated, unsafe x-ray equipment.

If identical prescriptions for the same medical treatment were allowed to vary as much, depending on which pharmacy filled them, there would be instant outcries of indignation, revocation of licenses, and, possibly, lawsuits. The likelihood of something like this happening is remote, however, as pharmacies and the pharmaceutical industry have a long history of competence and are closely watched by the FDA.

In comparison, the history of dental radiology is quite short and plagued with controversies. The effects of x-ray exposure may manifest themselves only many years after original exposure.

Years ago, for example, a number of dentists and dental x-ray technicians, apparently ignorant of the risk in radiology, suffered themselves from cancer of the hand as a result of holding the film or pointer cone during patient exposure. They eliminated this hazard by simply transferring it, asking the patient to hold the film in his mouth. But they did not solve the problem of *patient* overexposure.

Just as a pharmacist, in filling a prescription, must adhere strictly to the exact dosage prescribed, so should radiation be regulated and exposure limitations be enforced. Just as a small overdose of a potent drug may cost the patient's life, so may overexposure to radiation be deadly in the long run.

Much is said about average exposure for specific diagnostic x-rays, but no one ever mentions the wide variations that are prevalent today. Knowing what the *average* amount of radiation is for, say, a dental examination, can be of no consequence to the consumer who is, in fact, exposed to five times that average. The consumer must be educated about the potential health hazards versus health benefits of x-rays. He or she must also be encouraged to ask questions of those who administer the x-rays, about safety and exposure levels, instead of submitting blindly to any number of x-rays the dentist or physician may suggest. But most of all, the consumer should question the need for any given x-ray and always keep in mind that radiation is cumulative, which means that it increases in severity with repetition.

VI.

THE MISINFORMED CONSUMER

The American consumer is not being told the facts about dental x-ray overexposure. Information readily available to the general public is often misleading and incorrect. Unregulated secondhand machines are still in use in dental offices, though they may be the source of dangerous, unnecessary radiation of the vital organs in the head and neck area.

Used machines, of course, are less expensive than new ones. Therefore, they add to the profitability of a dental office. Unless government agencies control their use and safety, they will continue to be a threat to the health of dental patients.

Factual information concerning the dangers of dental x-rays is seldom disseminated by the news media. Professional publications for dentists give facts, but they are not readily accessible to the general public. Instead, the consumer is told a different story by government publications, newspaper articles, magazines, and radio or television — a story that always seems to contain the same deceptive language; namely, that dental x-ray exposures are very small and the danger is negligible. It is not surprising that the public is confused.

The FDA, in a 1976 publication concerning radiation control agencies,[27] stated that acceptable dental x-ray exposure ranges from 100 to 500 millirems per film. It also noted, without comment, that studies of x-ray examinations have shown exposures at skin level ranging from a low of 100 mR to 50 times as much, or 10 times higher than their stated acceptable limit of exposure.

In my opinion, the FDA should explain publicly if and why it is acceptable to them for dental x-ray exposure to vary so much for the same procedure, since it is known that there is a definite increase in risk involved in any increase in dosage.

There are dentists who disagree that dental x-ray exposure is low and harmless. For example, Loren F. Mills, DDS, a staff member at FDA, warned in a letter to the *Journal of the American Dental Association* (JADA)[32] that dental radiography requires relatively high exposures to critical areas of the head and neck, including "the red bone marrow of the mandible (jaw), the thyroid gland, and the lens of the eye."

Other professionals are also recognizing the danger. John W. Gofman, MD, for instance, in his recently published book, *Radiation and Human Health*, observes an association between dental x-rays and brain cancer.

Why, then, are there conflicting statements in consumer publications by the FDA, or publications which use FDA statistics? A consumer pamphlet[14] issued by the FDA claims rather ambiguously, "Less is known about the effects from *small* (emphasis added) amounts of radiation such as used in dental x-rays." This claim is repeated in JADA's 1982 consumer guide.

Despite the absence of data to support the claim, the *Los Angeles Times*, in an article headlined "Danger is Negligible in Dental X-Rays,"[33] quoted an FDA official in 1978 as saying that dental x-rays contribute only 3% of the total radiation from x-rays.

In 1979, *Glamour* magazine published a radiation exposure chart showing the range of dental x-ray examination doses to be from 10 to 30 mR.[34] *Good Housekeeping* printed the same figures quoting an FDA source.[35] Two years later, *Mademoiselle* also assured readers that dental x-rays give extremely low amounts of radiation.[36]

But the FDA states in its publication 76-8042[27] that dental x-ray exposure requires a minimum of 100 mR *per film* for a good radiograph. Radiation charts published in *Good Housekeeping* and *Glamour* magazines are deceiving the public when they give the complete examination dosage — which could require more than 10 films — as varying only between 10 and 30 millirems. To my inquiry concerning the accuracy of this chart, *Good Housekeeping* did not reply.

In 1981, WLS-TV, Chicago, published a pamphlet entitled "Seven On Your Side: X-Ray, The Unseen Danger." This pamphlet was also presented on the Phil Donahue Show and distributed nationwide. It gave grossly inaccurate x-ray exposure levels of 9 mR for complete dental examinations. The figure, it appears, came from a 1977 FDA publication chart titled, "Mean Active *Bone Marrow* (emphasis added) Dose to the Adult Population (1970)."[37]

It should be pointed out that an x-ray beam strikes the body with full force but has been reduced greatly in strength when it penetrates the bone marrow after passage through skin, flesh, and bone. Therefore, to use a bone marrow exposure level as an examination exposure level, which includes the skin, thyroid gland, eyes, brain, and bone marrow, is a serious distortion of fact.

The same FDA publication made it clear that a bone marrow dose of 2.9 mR compared with the average exposure at the skin of 1,110 mR for each dental film. It is hard to explain how the TV station staff could have overlooked that important point.

Again, it must be pointed out that bone marrow irradiation is associated with leukemia, but that there are various other cancers which could be induced by the *total* dose that is considerably higher than that mentioned in the pamphlet.

If repeated often enough to a large section of the population, statements such as these eventually convince the consumer that dental x-ray doses are so minimal that there is no cause for concern when undergoing x-ray examination.

Comparative data from *Nationwide Evaluation of X-Ray Trends Tabulations*, FDA, 1981 (see Appendix, page 56), indicate that median x-ray exposures from four out of nine medical procedures are considerably lower than the median exposure from dental procedures. Five other medical procedures expose patients to median levels higher than those in dental examinations. But not a single medical x-ray procedure, according to available FDA data, has a higher *maximum* exposure level than the dental bitewing examination (showing the upper and lower teeth on one film), which is an excessive 3,418 mR per film.

The FDA data clearly indicate that any x-ray examination, dental or medical, could expose the unsuspecting patient to considerable amounts of excess radiation, due to wide variations in dosage at different facilities. For example, they show that a chest x-ray could expose the patient to 1 mR* per film at one facility and 279 mR at another. The skull x-ray exposure could vary between 40 mR per film and 864; cervical spine, between 12 mR per film and 696; feet, between 5 mR per film and 534. (See Appendix, page 56, for additional data.) As far as dental x-rays are concerned, the exposure dosage for a dental periapical (showing the entire tooth, including the tip of the root) may vary between 49 mR per film and 2,825.

The maximum dental x-ray exposure could be about 10 times higher than the maximum chest x-ray exposure. Dental x-rays also irradiate very important organs of the head and neck. It is unfortunate that the majority of dentists, believing the myth that dental x-ray exposures are low, do not feel compelled to acquire up-to-date x-ray equipment.

---

*Unusually low exposure levels subject the patient to radiation without producing a satisfactory, good-quality radiograph, requiring more x-rays without any certainty that a good radiograph will be produced.

The unit prices for used x-ray equipment, I have been told, start at about $1,000, and for new, certified machines, at about $3,000.

At present, about 400 million dental x-rays are taken in the United States annually by 150,000 x-ray units, which amounts to an average of 2,666 x-ray films per unit a year. Assuming that the patient pays $4 per film, while the dentist's cost, including overhead, is approximately $2 per film, a profit of about $5,332 a year can be realized from one x-ray unit alone. If the unit cost is $1,000, this represents a 500% return on investment. That may be why some dentists invest in used x-ray equipment, which not only costs less than new machines but is also exempt from any regulations. Most of those outmoded x-ray units have not been improved with modern safety features, such as lead-lined, open-end cones to reduce scatter radiation; electronic timers to shorten exposure time to a fraction of a second; film-holding devices for better positioning; and proper filtration to remove harmful low energy x-rays from the beam.

In addition, these old machines are equipped with pointed plastic cones, which are not manufactured anymore, are not recommended by the American Dental Association, and are even outlawed in Illinois. They are the major source of secondary radiation that is considered as harmful as primary radiation itself. Secondary radiation, which could scatter in any direction, is difficult to measure. Therefore, dental x-ray exposures could be even higher than claimed. Yet, these cones continue to be widely used throughout the country on older machines.

The following sketch illustrates the two major sources of secondary radiation.

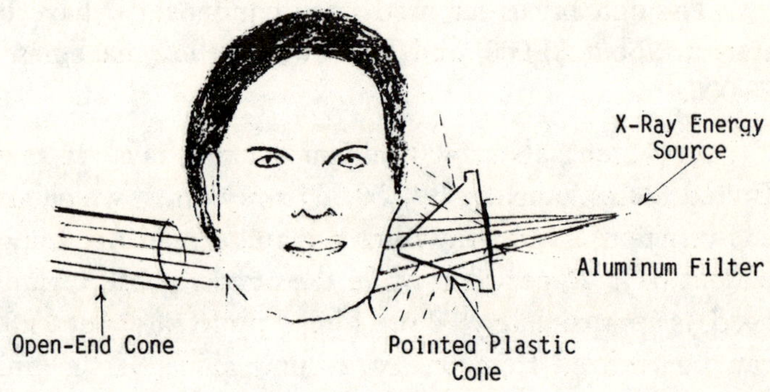

When the primary x-ray beam strikes the aluminum filter and pointed plastic cone, secondary radiation is produced. This radiation is hazardous not only to the patient but also to the operator. The open-end, lead-lined cone on newer machines eliminates this hazard.

Secondary radiation is also produced where the x-ray beam strikes the body (not shown in sketch). This action cannot be eliminated but can be reduced by keeping the radiation dose to the minimum needed to produce an acceptable radiograph.

VII.

LEGISLATIVE HISTORY
OF RADIATION CONTROL

As far as effective x-ray safeguards are concerned, the consumer stands almost alone, bearing most of the responsibility for his well-being in the face of profligate x-ray use, disingenuous regulations, and indifferent medical and dental establishments.

Congress was well aware of the fact that, in 1968, antiquated x-ray equipment was widely used in dental and medical offices. Therefore, when it passed the radiation control act, it also directed the Department of Health, Education, and Welfare to make a study concerning the need for controlling the sale of used, outmoded x-ray equipment, and to report the results of this study to Congress on or before January 1, 1970.[38]

In partial fulfillment of the department's responsibilities, the FDA made a limited study of the secondhand x-ray machine market in the United States in 1969, pertaining to the age and types of old x-ray equipment that has resale value; the size of the secondhand x-ray machine market; and purchase patterns involved in the sale of secondhand x-ray equipment.

This study did not contain any conclusions or recommendations, and no report was made to Congress concerning the results of the study (see Appendix, page 80). Therefore, it must be assumed that the responsibility — to report the results of this study to Congress — was not fulfilled. Consequently, no additional legislation was passed and existing legislation applies only to modern equipment. Used x-ray machines are still in operation without any safety controls.

It is obvious that a very important congressional mandate pertaining to old x-ray equipment was not carried out, and, as a result, many unsuspecting Americans are now subjected to dangerously high radiation exposure levels.

According to a 1968 Senate report,[2] a study showed that "approximately two-thirds of the estimated 112,000 medical x-ray machines surveyed did not meet current state recommendations or regulations."

This statement bears a striking resemblance to a similar revelation made 14 years later on a TV program in Los Angeles, "Wide-range violations per x-ray machine are rampant throughout the country." Nevertheless, in the JADA's guide, the consumer is led to believe that regulations of x-ray equipment provide a sound measure of radiation protection.

This is one of those unsubstantiated statements that only confuse the consumer and is contradicted by the nationwide surveys of x-ray equipment showing a wide variation of exposures due to the lack of regulation.

The government is responsible for protecting the consumer against manufacture and sale of hazardous household appliances. But the sale of unsafe, secondhand x-ray equipment (equally if not more hazardous) is legal and flourishing. It is time the consumer is protected against this danger, too.

In conclusion, it is appropriate to refer to a statement made in 1973 before the Senate Committee of Commerce by Edward I. Koch, then a New York congressman and later mayor of New York City. What he said is as true today as it was then when Congress was considering a bill that would have required *all* x-ray machines to meet the same standards. That bill did not pass, and no progress has been made in the intervening decade.

Congressman Koch testified that, since he had been advised it was feasible to upgrade old machines to meet the new standards, there seemed to be "no valid reason" for not doing so. The average life span of an x-ray machine, he had been advised, was 15 to 20 years, with some lasting as long as 40 years. He also referred to an estimated replacement rate of 5%.

The chief of radiation control in New York had estimated that 50% of the x-ray equipment sold in the city was secondhand, according to Koch. A survey of 765 of the resold units had identified 595 deficiencies. "No individual," he summed up, "should be required to submit to x-radiation by a machine which does not meet the established performance standards."

His 1973 projection of a 5% annual replacement rate proved to be wrong, however. By 1982, eight years after the federal performance standard had been implemented, about 20% of all x-ray equipment was new and certified. This means that each year only about 2½% of old x-ray equipment is replaced with new, certified machines, and all other units traded are secondhand.

For his own protection, the consumer must avoid those medical and dental facilities that use pre-1974 x-ray equipment. The only way he can do this is by acquiring a list of facilities that use modern, certified machines. Such a list is available from the U.S. Bureau of Radiological Health, Food and Drug Administration, Rockville, Maryland 20857, for a fee.

Before submitting to an x-ray examination, the consumer should ascertain that (a) the x-ray equipment is federally certified as meeting the 1974 performance standard; (b) the x-ray machine operator is qualified; and (c) authentic x-ray exposure data for that machine are available upon request.

APPENDIX

The Cancer Risk Nobody Dares to Talk About

RUN DATE: WEDNESDAY MAY 13, 1981   NATIONWIDE EVALUATION OF X-RAY TRENDS   PAGE:
                             TABLE: WEIGHTED MEDIAN INDEXES BY TYPE OF EXAM/PROJECTION
                        THIS TABLE INCLUDES ALL DATA FROM THE REPRESENTATIVE CATEGORY ONLY.

STATE: ALL STATES DATA ONLY
DATE INTERVALS: FROM 01/01/80 TO 12/31/80

			OVARIAN DOSE INDEX (MRAD)	TESTICULAR DOSE INDEX (MRAD)	EXPOSURE AT SKIN ENTRANCE (MR)	SURFACE EXPOSURE INTEGRAL (R X SQ CM)	RED BONE MARROW DOSE INDEX (MRAD)	THYROID DOSE INDEX (MRAD)
CHEST (P/A)		MINIMUM VALUE	<.5	<.5	1.	1.	<.5	<.5
		1ST QUARTILE	<.5	<.5	12.	13.	1.	<.5
ALL STATES		MEDIAN	<.5	<.5	17.	20.	2.	1.
NO. OF SURVEYS	816	3RD QUARTILE	<.5	<.5	26.	29.	3.	1.
		MAXIMUM VALUE	7.	1.	279.	390.	18.	6.
SKULL (LATERAL)		MINIMUM VALUE	<.5	<.5	40.	11.	1.	<.5
		1ST QUARTILE	<.5	<.5	105.	38.	3.	10.
ALL STATES		MEDIAN	<.5	<.5	154.	85.	5.	24.
NO. OF SURVEYS	79	3RD QUARTILE	<.5	<.5	240.	132.	8.	70.
		MAXIMUM VALUE	<.5	<.5	864.	841.	26.	170.
ABD. (KUB)(A/P)		MINIMUM VALUE	11.	<.5	48.	29.	1.	<.5
		1ST QUARTILE	78.	4.	375.	252.	11.	<.5
ALL STATES		MEDIAN	107.	7.	485.	376.	16.	<.5
NO. OF SURVEYS	473	3RD QUARTILE	163.	12.	698.	565.	26.	<.5
		MAXIMUM VALUE	478.	271.	2359.	1962.	79.	<.5
RETR. PYELO. (A/P)		MINIMUM VALUE	17.	<.5	89.	55.	1.	<.5
		1ST QUARTILE	112.	6.	475.	346.	18.	<.5
ALL STATES		MEDIAN	120.	8.	638.	533.	18.	<.5
NO. OF SURVEYS	66	3RD QUARTILE	156.	11.	829.	627.	24.	<.5
		MAXIMUM VALUE	559.	364.	2257.	1231.	64.	<.5
THOR. SPINE (A/P)		MINIMUM VALUE	<.5	<.5	90.	51.	2.	2.
		1ST QUARTILE	<.5	<.5	295.	198.	10.	14.
ALL STATES		MEDIAN	<.5	<.5	405.	270.	14.	14.
NO. OF SURVEYS	27	3RD QUARTILE	<.5	<.5	485.	413.	15.	33.
		MAXIMUM VALUE	4.	<.5	980.	493.	20.	282.
CERVICAL SPINE (A/P)		MINIMUM VALUE	<.5	<.5	12.	6.	<.5	10.
		1ST QUARTILE	<.5	<.5	57.	20.	1.	38.
ALL STATES		MEDIAN	<.5	<.5	130.	45.	2.	89.
NO. OF SURVEYS	84	3RD QUARTILE	<.5	<.5	207.	69.	2.	151.
		MAXIMUM VALUE	<.5	<.5	696.	768.	17.	558.
LUM-SAC SPINE (A/P)		MINIMUM VALUE	10.	<.5	65.	27.	1.	<.5
		1ST QUARTILE	95.	6.	455.	289.	13.	<.5
ALL STATES		MEDIAN	126.	9.	622.	408.	19.	<.5
NO. OF SURVEYS	578	3RD QUARTILE	181.	14.	796.	531.	26.	<.5
		MAXIMUM VALUE	775.	270.	3040.	4130.	136.	2.
FULL SPINE (A/P)		MINIMUM VALUE	6.	<.5	60.	117.	2.	32.
		1ST QUARTILE	53.	2.	235.	515.	18.	193.
ALL STATES		MEDIAN	111.	3.	486.	1071.	40.	335.
NO. OF SURVEYS	28	3RD QUARTILE	184.	6.	708.	1261.	62.	574.
		MAXIMUM VALUE	230.	15.	1061.	1560.	67.	745.
FEET (D/P)		MINIMUM VALUE	***	***	5.	2.	***	***
		1ST QUARTILE	***	***	8.	4.	***	***
ALL STATES		MEDIAN	***	***	106.	58.	***	***
NO. OF SURVEYS	36	3RD QUARTILE	***	***	327.	279.	***	***
		MAXIMUM VALUE	***	***	534.	510.	***	***
DENTAL B.W. POST		MINIMUM VALUE	***	***	41.	1.	***	***
		1ST QUARTILE	***	***	227.	7.	***	***
ALL STATES		MEDIAN	***	***	310.	9.	***	***
NO. OF SURVEYS	1036	3RD QUARTILE	***	***	425.	13.	***	***
		MAXIMUM VALUE	***		➡ 3418.	136.	***	***
DENTAL PERIAPICAL		MINIMUM VALUE	***	***	49.	2.	***	***
		1ST QUARTILE	***	***	245.	7.	***	***
ALL STATES		MEDIAN	***	***	289.	11.	***	***
NO. OF SURVEYS	321	3RD QUARTILE	***	➡ ***	404.	13.	***	***
		MAXIMUM VALUE	***		➡ 2825.	76.	***	***

December 30, 1980

Mr. J. Arthur Lazell
Assistant Director
Bureau of Radiological Health
Food and Drug Administration
Rockville, Maryland 20857

Dear Mr. Lazell:

Thank you very much for your recent informative letter
and the enclosed publications concerning the reduction of
mammographic exposures in the United States.

I would appreciate obtaining additional information
about the number of mammographic units in the United States
that have been certified as meeting the DHEW Diagnostic
X-ray Standard.

Thank you for your courtesy.

Sincerely,

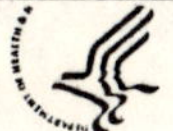

DEPARTMENT OF HEALTH & HUMAN SERVICES   Public Health Service

---

Food and Drug Administration
Rockville MD 20857

January 15, 1980 (1981)

Ref: F81-736

Mr. Bruno Barmus

Dear Mr. Barmus:

Mr. Lazell has been out of the office this week because of illness so

I am responding to your request to avoid delay. As requested in your

letter dated December 30, 1980, 727 mammographic units have been

certified as meeting the Food and Drug Administration performance

standard for diagnostic x-ray equipment. I hope this information is

helpful.

Sincerely yours,

Virginia R. Watterson
Secretary to:
J. Arthur Lazell
Assistant Director

THE CANCER RISK NOBODY DARES TO TALK ABOUT

April 5, 1979

Mr. Joseph E. Ward, Chief
Department of Health Services
Radiologic Health Section
555 Capitol Mall
Sacramento, CA 95814

Dear Mr. Ward:

Mr. Califano, Secretary of Health, Education and Welfare, on nation-wide T.V. on April 4, 1979 stated that: chest x-ray exposes the patient to 40 mR. and dental x-ray to 70 mR.

I would like to know the x-ray radiation doses (minimum and maximum) in California for dental and chest x-rays.

1977 CALIF.

PA CHEST

MINIMUM	5 mR
MAXIMUM	92 mR
MEAN	22.3 mR

PERIAPICAL (DENTAL)

MINIMUM	45 mR
MAXIMUM	4106 mR
MEAN	478.6 mR

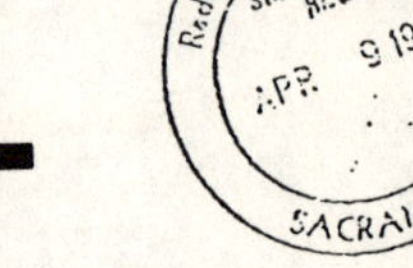

APPENDIX

a·practitioner's guide to the diagnostic x-ray equipment standard

EXCERPTS from HEW Publication (FDA) 78-8050, February 1978

MAJOR PROVISIONS OF THE STANDARD

Two general points should be made about the standard at the outset. First, it is an equipment performance standard. It cannot require equipment design features. A certain type of beam-limiting device, for example, cannot be stipulated. It is up to the manufacturer to determine how to achieve levels of equipment performance mandated by the standard.

The other point is that the standard does not regulate diagnostic x-ray equipment users. It neither requires health professionals to practice radiology in certain ways nor prohibits them from using x-ray equipment for a desired purpose. 

The standard applies to major components, as well as complete systems, manufactured after August 1, 1974. With respect to systems in use prior to the effective date, it in no way requires or implies that these units *must* be modified, upgraded, or discarded. 

UPGRADING USED EQUIPMENT

The question of upgrading equipment not made under the standard has concerned the Food and Drug Administration, as well as the Congress where legislation has been introduced to require improved radiation protection capability in used x-ray machines. In 1973, FDA proposed an interpretation of the intent of the Radiation Control for Health and

Safety Act regulations as requiring used x-ray equipment refurbished, rebuilt, or reassembled after August 1, 1974 to comply with the standard for new equipment. The proposal was later modified, however, because of the possibility that it might cause shortages of acceptable used equipment and thus adversely affect health care. 

In the end, the regulations were amended to effect a more gradual upgrading of equipment by:

- Requiring that an x-ray system made before August 1, 1974 that is altered by installation of a certified component, will thereafter have to use only certified replacement components. This provision was needed to prevent the degradation of certified systems by the installation of noncertified components.

- Prohibiting the assembly of uncertified components into systems reassembled and sold after August 1, 1979—5 years after the standard's effective date. Components not certified under the standard will have to be replaced in such systems.

The 5-year grace period for application of the standard to reassembled equipment allows time for adequate inventories of *certified components* to be produced. Furthermore, the period conforms with estimates of the approximate time it will take certified equipment to move into the used x-ray market from hospital radiology departments and other high workload facilities. /4

<u>EXCERPTS</u>

HEARINGS

BEFORE THE

<u>COMMITTEE ON COMMERCE</u> UNITED STATES SENATE

ON

Public Law 90–602

RADIATION CONTROL FOR HEALTH AND SAFETY ACT OF 1968

MARCH 8, 9, AND 12, 1973

STATEMENT OF JOHN C. VILLFORTH, DIRECTOR, BUREAU OF
RADIOLOGICAL HEALTH, FOOD AND DRUG ADMINISTRATION,
DEPARTMENT OF HEALTH, EDUCATION, AND WELFARE

One of the more significant accomplishments of the Bureau took place on August 15, 1972, with the final publication of a performance standard for "Diagnostic X-ray Systems and their Major Components." This standard becomes effective August 15, 1973. Of the four class-type equipment performance standards developed to date, the diagnostic X-ray equipment standard is by far the most complex, and far-reaching in its impact on the public's heath. Its development required 2 years of concentrated effort by a considerable part of the Bureau's scientific, engineering, and technical staff. An extensive effort on the part of the FDA has been budgeted to administer this standard and assure compliance with its provisions.

This standard is important inasmuch as 90 percent of the public's exposure to all types of manmade radiation comes from diagnostic X-radiation used in the healing arts.

REPORT BY THE Comptroller General

OF THE UNITED STATES

Radiation Control Programs
Provide Limited Protection

HRD-80-25
DECEMBER 4, 1979

The programs involve BRH analysis of information recorded on dosimetry cards. The State mails the cards to X-ray facilities, where the cards are exposed to radiation and returned to the State. The State then mails the cards to BRH, which reads and evaluates the data and reports the results to the State. <u>Since the programs began, 38 States surveyed 35,224 dental units. BRH's analysis indicated that exposures from 12,680 units appeared excessively high.</u>  <u>Forty-five States surveyed 3,253 mammographic units, resulting in BRH identifying 1,496 units with either excessively high or unusually low X-ray exposure.</u> 1/

1/Unusually low exposure could result in an additional X-ray
   to get an acceptable picture.

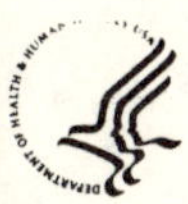

DEPARTMENT OF HEALTH & HUMAN SERVICES   Public Health Service

Food and Drug Administration
Rockville MD 20857

APR 12 1982

Mr. Bruno Barmus

Dear Mr. Barmus:

As I mentioned in my March 2 letter to you, your letter of February 10 to Secretary Schweiker was referred to the Bureau of Radiological Health for reply. Because of the background surrounding your letter, I have personally reviewed it and your enclosures. I have also reviewed the entire file of correspondence (summary table enclosed) which Bureau of Radiological Health (BRH) staff have had with you since 1978.

My review reveals three themes which recur throughout your correspondence: first, that there is inadequate regulation of used x-ray machines; second, that government should set exposure limits for x-ray examinations; and third, that we have denied the existence of variations in exposure among different medical and dental radiology facilities. Several letters contained requests for materials or information in addition to assertions of inadequate government attention to the problem of over-exposure to x rays. I find that my staff has prepared 20 replies to your inquiries and concerns during the last 39 months.

Mr. Barmus, apparently we have been unable to convey to you an understanding of the limitations of our statutory authority, nor have we been able to suitably describe the rationale for our programs to control unnecessary population exposure to medical and dental radiation. As we have previously described, the Bureau has programs aimed at (1) ensuring that radiation-emitting electronic devices are properly manufactured and assembled; (2) educating professionals in proper use of radiation-emitting products; and (3) educating consumers to take an active role in reducing unnecessary radiation exposure. Our statutory authority provides explicit limits to what we can do to implement these goals. Details about our authority and publications from many of our programs have been shared with you during the exchange of letters between you and BRH staff. Let me reiterate. By law we are only permitted to regulate the manufacture and assembly of new x-ray units. We have no authority to force individuals to use the equipment in prescribed ways. Individual States may require certain practices within their borders, but that power does not extend to the Federal Government. In what follows, I have attempted to address your three major concerns. Regarding your assertion that we have denied the existence of variation in exposure among different medical and dental radiology facilities, it is interesting that the figures you quote to demonstrate such variance are from BRH publications. This information is a

Page 2 - Mr. Bruno Barmus

matter of public record. The information has been distributed nationwide. I have used the information in testimony before Congress on many occasions. The evidence is clear that we have not attempted to obscure the fact that radiation exposures vary from facility to facility and, indeed, from patient to patient.

Because of the existence of such variation, the Bureau has for some time promoted cooperative programs with State radiological health agencies to reduce that variance. We shared with you information from our DENT (Dental Exposure Normalization Technique) program. That program has been successful in reducing the variance among participating dental x-ray facilities. But that variance cannot be reduced to zero. No program can do that. There are too many factors that affect patient exposure and dose to make that possible. However, the film manufacturers, the dental profession, the State health agencies and ourselves are all engaged in activities to reduce the exposure from dental x-ray procedures to as low a figure that is consistent with a useful x-ray examination. I've included some information which shows the extent of dental x-ray exposure reduction that has occurred over the past several years.

You have expressed a concern over the use of used or old x-ray equipment. The Bureau has thoroughly investigated the issues surrounding the used x-ray equipment problem. Our 1978 analysis on the issue was presented to a statutorily required committee of industrial and consumer representatives. It was published for comment in the Federal Register (copy enclosed), and was reviewed by numerous individuals and organizations. The bottom line on that analysis is that the remedies available to us under our current statutory authority are not cost-effective for addressing potential problems with individual assemblies of older equipment. State regulatory authority and the marketplace, itself, were identified as more effective mechanisms for achieving the desired end. I should note that the analysis was performed with respect to medical x-ray units. The benefits specified in the report would be significantly lower for dental units and, therefore, make the argument to regulate the sale of used dental equipment even less cost-effective.

In order to clarify what we can and cannot do with respect to assuring the radiation safety of older equipment, let me outline the limitations of our statutory and regulatory authority:

(1) For equipment manufactured prior to October 18, 1968, FDA has
      authority under the Food, Drug and Cosmetic Act to declare
      such equipment mislabeled or misbranded if it does not meet
      the manufacturer's claims or advertized specifications.
      Manufacturers must correct flaws in such products or the
      equipment can be seized and impounded.

Page 3 - Mr. Bruno Barmus

    (2)   For x-ray equipment manufactured after October 18, 1968, FDA has authority under the Radiation Control for Health and Safety Act of 1968 to declare a defect on such equipment. That is, manufacturers can be forced to correct excessive x-ray emissions if such emissions can be related to a design or production error by the manufacturer. This authority does not apply to excess emissions of radiation caused by poor operator techniques.

    (3)   Diagnostic x-ray equipment manufactured after August 1, 1974, must be certified as meeting the diagnostic x-ray equipment performance standard. Part of this standard addresses the "remanufacture" or reassembly of old equipment, but only if that equipment changes ownership and is moved to a new location. It does not apply to the equipment that concerns you.

    (4)   For x-ray equipment manufactured after July 17, 1979, FDA has authority under the Medical Device Amendments of 1976 to ban the use of such equipment if it presents a substantial risk of illness or injury.

As you can see, all of these authorities refer to manufacturer-related problems. None of these regulatory remedies can legally be applied in the case that you have brought to our attention (i.e., excessive exposure caused by poor operator technique).

As I mentioned earlier, there are many parameters under the control of the operator and the practitioner which have a greater bearing on patient exposure and dose than the age of the x-ray machine. Our experience indicates that age of equipment is far less important than the training, supervision, and practices of the personnel operating the machine. A new machine can give far too much exposure if improperly adjusted or if incorrect settings are utilized. Likewise, an older machine can give good radiographs with very acceptable exposures when properly maintained and utilized. In any case, the radiation control agencies in each State have the authority and responsibility for inspecting x-ray equipment of any age and for assuring its compliance with State regulations.

In reviewing the file of correspondence, Mr. Barmus, I noted that you have corresponded with the radiologic health section of the California Department of Health. Mr. England from that department provided you with copies of the radiation control regulations of California. It appears you may have misunderstood the section of those regulations that deals with used equipment. It states "Any existing machine or installation need not be replaced or substan-

Page 4 - Mr. Bruno Barnus

tially modified to conform to the requirements of this regulation <u>provided that the user demonstrates to the Department's satisfaction achievement of equivalent protection through other means</u>" (emphasis added). That section requires that existing x-ray equipment, that is, equipment manufactured before July 31, 1974, must meet the equivalent level of protection as that afforded by equipment manufactured after the July date. Again, the fact that an older x-ray unit may have had a higher exposure reading at the Goodley Professional Dental Corporation, is not an indictment of the equipment itself. Operator technique is a more likely explanation. You'll recall that Dr. Miller called attention to the Goodley problem in his April 5, 1979, letter to the California State Board of Dental Examiners.

Finally, you have suggested that we mandate exposure limits for various x-ray procedures. The Bureau does not have the statutory authority to do so. We are fully aware that this has been attempted in a few States, but the effectiveness of this approach has not been established. It is not at all clear that a significant amount of unneccessary exposure is reduced by establishing such a limit. In addition, to be effective, such limits must be enforced, and enforcement is exceedingly difficult and expensive. Without enforcement, the effectiveness of such limits is questionable. However, the whole issue of exposure limits has not yet been resolved in the States, and it is possible that this approach might become more widely adopted.

As we have pointed out before, consumers such as yourself can take a number of measures to help avoid unnecessary medical and dental x-ray exposure. These have been widely publicized in our consumer education materials copies of which have previously been sent to you. We are encouraging consumers to talk to their doctor or dentist, and tell him/her about their radiological health concerns. An increasing number of doctors and dentists are eager to share information about their procedures and answer your questions. For example, I've included with this letter, a copy of a recent publication by the American Dental Association which presents that organization's position on patient protection and rights in dental radiology. By doing these things, consumers not only gain information, but also encourage continued vigilance by the practitioner. Of course, if a person is not satisfied with the responses or attitudes of the practitioner on radiological issues or other health care matters, he/she has the right to seek another practitioner.

It is our intent to always be responsive to those who write to us. My review of the correspondence between BRH and you indicates that we have addressed all your concerns on numerous occasions. I regret that we have been unsuccessful in communicating to you the merits of our programs and the depth of our commit-

Page 5 - Mr. Bruno Barmus

ment to the goal of protecting the public health. Hopefully, the impact of our programs in the future will be adequate testimony of our dedication.

Sincerely yours,

John C. Villforth
Director
Bureau of Radiological Health

Enclosures

The Cancer Risk Nobody Dares to Talk About

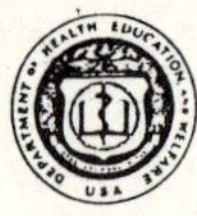

DEPARTMENT OF HEALTH, EDUCATION, AND WELFARE
PUBLIC HEALTH SERVICE
FOOD AND DRUG ADMINISTRATION
ROCKVILLE, MARYLAND 20857

January 8, 1979

Mr. Bruno Barmus

Dear Mr. Barmus:

Your letter to Commissioner Kennedy concerning radiation hazards in dental
x rays has been referred to my office for reply.

Your concern about the use of unnecessary dental x rays is shared by the
government and as you point out in your letter the FDA is committed to
improving communication by educating consumers about the benefits and risks
of diagnostic x rays. Radiographs are one of the most important diagnostic
aids the dentist has to detect hidden cavities and other problems that can
affect dental health. The periodic use of x rays during dental checkup
enables the dentist to detect conditions that, if left untreated, would
eventually affect the function and appearance of your teeth. Early treatment may save money, but, more important, it saves teeth. However, x rays
should not be taken routinely, but only after the dentist has done an oral
examination and taken a medical and dental history. Then, if the dentist
determines x rays are necessary, they may be taken. The decision to use
x rays must be made by the dentist, based upon the general and dental health
needs of the patient. The primary deciding factor is the welfare of the
patient. The nature and extent of actual or suspected disease and its
response to treatment constitute the only rational basis for determining the
need or the frequency of dental x-ray examinations.

Dental x-ray equipment is not considered to be a major factor in unnecessary
radiation exposure today. While the Federal performance standard took
effect August 1, 1974, manufacturers were aware of the requirements several
years before and x-ray equipment manufactured during that period of time
essentially meets the Federal performance standard. As a matter of fact,
most of the dental x-ray equipment manufactured after approximately 1955
are reported to be in compliance with State regulations. While we do not
recommend the use of pointed plastic cones its really a minor source of
secondary radiation and should be of no major concern. The Bureau of
Radiological Health has recently dropped a proposal to regulate open-ended
position aiming devices because data indicated that if they were used with
the bisected-angle technique, the radiation dosage could be higher than
when a pointed plastic cone is used.

Page -2- Mr. Bruno Barmus

The Bureau of Radiological Health in cooperation with State and local
health departments has been conducting a program called Dental Exposure
Normalization Technique (DENT) to reduce unnecessary exposure to x rays
and to improve the quality of dental radiographs. DENT recommends that
dental exposures should be in the 200-500 mR per film range, depending
upon the kilovoltage the dentist uses. The State of California is pres-
ently participating in this program. It will take them approximately
five years to survey all the dental offices and to visit the offices that
need corrections.

For your information I am enclosing the following articles:

1. Recommendations in radiographic practices - March 1978
2. Safe use of medical x rays
3. We want you to know about diagnostic x rays
4. Radiation and Health

We appreciate your interest in radiological health and if I can be of any
further assistance, please do not hesitate to contact me.

Sincerely yours,

James W. Miller, D.D.S., M.S.
Assistant Director for Dentistry
Bureau of Radiological Health

Enclosures (4)

The Cancer Risk Nobody Dares to Talk About

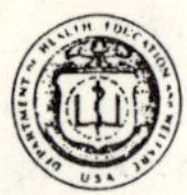

DEPARTMENT OF HEALTH, EDUCATION, AND WELFARE
PUBLIC HEALTH SERVICE
FOOD AND DRUG ADMINISTRATION
ROCKVILLE, MARYLAND 20857

February 16, 1979

Dear Mr. Barmus

I appreciate your concern that some dental offices use more radiation than
necessary when taking x-rays. While the practice in itself may not cause
any demonstrable effect, it is unnecessary radiation which should be eliminated. I cannot defend the practice, nor is it condoned by any other
agency or professional group. The problem in dentistry is generally not
with equipment but how the equipment is used by personnel in the dental
office. This needless to say is difficult to regulate and an area in which
we have no authority. User control has traditionally been the responsibility
of the State. However, we are aware that it is a problem which we would
like to remedy and have tried to correct the situation in two ways. One,
is by working with States, trying to assist them, within our limited resources to deal with the problem. Our major current effort to assure that
dental exposures per film are within a recommended range is the DENT program
which I mentioned in my previous letter to you. To date thirty-eight States
have cooperated with us in this effort. California is one of the States.
Unfortunately California has over 18,000 dental x-ray machines in the State
and very few resources to visit dental offices identified by DENT as using
more radiation than necessary. Just advising the dentist by letter does
not seem to take care of the problem, his entire procedure should be checked
to determine where the problem lies. This requires trained people who may
not be available due to budget or other constraints on the radiation control
agencies.

The other approach is educational, directed at the dental profession both in
school and in practice. Our goal is to have only knowledgeable and qualified
individuals prescribing and taking radiographs. We have developed a variety
of educational and training materials and programs to improve the skills of
the dentist and dental assistants. We are working with the appropriate
National and local professional societies, and the schools to communicate
to dentistry what should be known about radiological health. We feel that
we have had considerable success with this approach but it is apparent that
we still have a way to go.

In dental radiology the schools determine what is taught and how well. State
Dental Boards of Examiners determine who is qualified to take dental x-rays
and by what criteria. Without authority to regulate the competency that an

[68]

individual must demonstrate before prescribing or subjecting humans to
x-ray procedures, radiation control agencies are limited to the role
of an advisor only. Fortunately the bulk of the dental profession I
believe is concerned and is trying to limit the amount of radiation
their patients receive. Unfortunately there are those who through
ignorance or indifference do not follow recommended practices. These
we are trying to reach through avenues currently available to us.

Your continued interest in this matter is appreciated. I am making a
copy of your letter and my reply available to the California Department
of Health Services. Hopefully they can expedite their visit to the
Goodley Professional Dental Corporation to rectify the apparent over-use
of radiation.

Sincerely yours,

James W. Miller, D.D.S.
Assistant Director for Dentistry
Office of Health Affairs
Bureau of Radiological Health

cc:
Dr. Donald Kennedy, FDA
Mr. Joseph Ward, CA State Rep.
Mr. Morgan Seal, Reg. 1X, FDA
Mr. Robert Eccleston, BRH
Dr. O. Johnson, BRH
Dr. L. Crabtree, BRH

CALIFORNIA
(Excerpts)

RADIATION CONTROL

REGULATIONS

Reprinted from the

California Administrative Code

Title 17. Health

TITLE 17   RADIATION   539
(Register 76, No. 35—8-28-76)

Group 3. Standards for Protection Against Radiation

Article 1. General

30252. Scope. This regulation applies to all persons who possess sources of radiation, except as exempt from the licensing and registration requirements or otherwise specifically exempted by the provisions of Group 1 and Group 2 of this subchapter. The provisions of the following listed sections shall not apply with respect to patients during intentional exposure to radiation for the purpose of medical or dental diagnosis or medical therapy: 30265, 30276, 30277, 30280, 30295, 30297.

30295. Notification of Incidents. (a) Immediate Notification.

30297. Reports of Overexposures and Excessive Levels and Concentrations.

30305. General Provisions.
(a) (1) This article pertains to use of X-rays in medicine, dentistry, osteopathy, chiropractic, podiatry, and veterinary medicine. The provisions of this article are in addition to, and not in substitution for, other applicable provisions of this regulation and of Group 1 of this subchapter.
(2) Any existing machine or installation need not be replaced or substantially modified to conform to the requirements of this regulation provided that the user demonstrates to the Department's satisfaction achievement of equivalent protection through other means.

(4) For X-ray equipment manufactured after July 31, 1974, the user shall provide sufficient maintenance to keep the equipment in compliance with all applicable radiation protection sections of the Code of Federal Regulations, Title 21, Chapter 1, Subchapter J, Part 1020, Sections 1020.30, 1020.31, and 1020.32.

DEPARTMENT OF HEALTH
714-744 P STREET
SACRAMENTO, CALIFORNIA 95814
(916) 445-6695

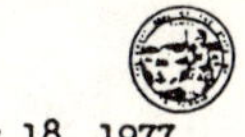

October 18, 1977

Mr. Bruno Barmus

████████████████████████

Dear Mr. Barmus:

Your letter of October 6, 1977 regarding the use of dental X-rays has been forwarded to my attention. However, our program deals only with the registration and inspection of dental X-ray equipment and in some instances the certification of persons to administer and use X-rays on humans. Dentists are specifically exempted from our jurisdiction. 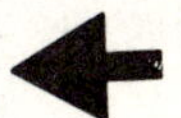

The very relevant questions you have raised are more appropriately addressed under the Dental Practice Act and not the rules and regulations governing our program. Accordingly, I have forwarded your letter to the Board of Dental Examiners and asked that they research and respond to your inquiry.

Thank you for your concern in this matter and I am certain the Board will be contacting you in the very near future.

Sincerely,

John J. Kearns
Senior Health Physicist
Certification
Radiologic Health Section

November 29, 1977

With reference to your letter of November 23, 1977, our records are not kept in a manner to provide the information you requested regarding the names of dentists in the Los Angeles area who have up-to-date equipment complete with electronic timer and devices for holding intra-oral films. 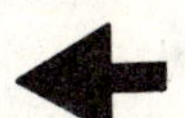

It should be noted that Section 30311. (a) (5) of the California Radiation Control Regulations requires that a device be provided to terminate the exposure after a pre-set time or exposure on all dental radiographic equipment. However, there is no requirement regarding the use of a device to hold the intra-oral film during exposure.

I trust the Board of Dental Examiners has responded to your earlier letter, but if I can be of further assistance, please feel free to contact me.

Sincerely,

John J. Kearns
Senior Health Physicist
Certification
Radiologic Health Section

THE CANCER RISK NOBODY DARES TO TALK ABOUT

August 25, 1978

Dear Mr. Barmus

I am in receipt of your letter of August 14, 1978, and have reviewed your previous request for this refund.

Our records show that on your September 20 appointment, you were not given an examination because of your refusal to have X-rays taken. However, you did have your teeth cleaned at that time. The charge for prophylaxis (cleaning) as of that date was $25. Had you had the X-rays and diagnosis, the charge would have been an additional $15. The $25 you paid was the correct amount for the services performed. We billed your insurance company for the $25, and they sent us a check for $16 which we forwarded to you.

You certainly have the right to decline having X-rays taken, Mr. Barmus but as we explained in a previous letter; our technicians and facilities meet all California standards for safety and competence. X-rays permit the doctor to detect dental problems at the best time for treatment--before they are large enough to be visible upon examination. This can prevent a great deal of expense and discomfort for our patients.

I hope that this explanation clears up the matter for you. If you have any further questions, please feel free to contact us.

Sincerely,

DEPARTMENT OF HEALTH SERVICES
714-744 P STREET
SACRAMENTO, CALIFORNIA 95814

(916) 445-6256

September 7, 1978

Per your telephone request, the thermoluminescence dosimeter (TLD) readings of exposures from the dental X-ray machines located at

are as follows:

X-ray Unit	Date Exposed	kVp	mA	Timer Setting	mR/film (bite wing)
Ritter Room 2	1/27/76	65	5	1 sec	620
Ritter Room 4	1/27/76	65	5	1 sec	619
Oralix Rooms 10 & 12	1/27/76	50	5	1 sec	1735

These readings were obtained from TLD cards exposed by the registrant according to instructions given in the enclosed Form RH 4097.

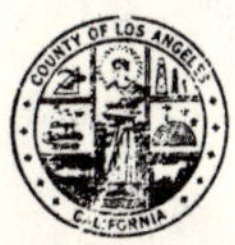

COUNTY OF LOS ANGELES - DEPARTMENT OF HEALTH SERVICES

313 NORTH FIGUEROA STREET ● LOS ANGELES, CALIFORNIA 90012 ● PHONE

Morrison E. Chamberlin
Director
974-8104

Robert L. Spears, M.D.
Acting Medical Director
974-8106

HEALTH SERVICES
PREVENTIVE HEALTH
HOSPITALS
MENTAL HEALTH
COMPARATIVE VETERINARY
MEDICINE

REGIONS

CENTRAL

Deputy Director
1100 N. MISSION ROAD
LOS ANGELES 90033
PHONE 213-226-6421

COASTAL

DONALD W. AVANT
Deputy Director
1401 CHESTNUT AVENUE
LONG BEACH 90813
PHONE 213-775-7401

SAN FERNANDO-
ANTELOPE VALLEY

DORRIS M HARRIS, M D
Deputy Director
7533 VAN NUYS BOULEVARD
ROOM 400, SOUTH TOWER
VAN NUYS 91405
PHONE 213-997-1800

SAN GABRIEL VALLEY

ALVIN KARP
Deputy Director
1435 WEST COVINA PARKWAY
WEST COVINA 91790
PHONE 213-338-8461

SOUTHEAST

MELVIN J FLEMING
Deputy Director
12020 COMPTON AVENUE
LOS ANGELES 90059
PHONE 213-636-0961

TO: SUPERVISOR EDMUND D. EDELMAN

FROM: MORRISON E. CHAMBERLIN, DIRECTOR
     DEPARTMENT OF HEALTH SERVICES

DATE: FEBRUARY 6, 1978

SUBJECT: CONCERN ABOUT RADIATION SAFETY IN
     DENTAL X-RAY FACILITIES

This is in response to your letter of January 11, 1978 addressed
to Assemblyman Mike Roos requesting reports on the matter of
information and standards applicable to the safe use of dental
x-ray equipment. This Department, through the Radiation
Management Office, is currently responsible for and conducting
a program of radiation safety and control throughout the County
of Los Angeles. This program enforces the requirements of the
California Radiation Control Regulations, Title 17, California
Administrative Code. The purpose of the regulations is to minimize exposure to the general population and the worker. The
regulations include standards of safety applicable to all types
of radiation facilities including dental x-ray offices.

Under a contract which the County has with the State Department
of Health, all x-ray facilities in the County of Los Angeles
are periodically inspected to insure compliance with legal
standards. This activity has been carried out in the County
of Los Angeles (as well as throughout California) for over ten
years. During this period, essentially all dental x-ray facilities
have received comprehensive inspections, and many have been checked
several times. In addition to the inspectional activities, in-
vestigations and surveys of incidents or other concerns occurring
in dental x-ray facilities have been made by Radiation Management
staff with appropriate corrective action required through issuance
of legal citations.

As changes develop in the field of dental x-ray technology, improvements are made in the inspectional technique and procedure.
An example of such change is a current program measuring the
radiation output of dental x-ray machines throughout the State for
the purpose of reducing radiation exposure of patients to the low-
est possible level. Radiation specialists of this Department make
visits to assist dentists using machines with excessive radiation
to achieve the maximum possible reduction of x-ray consistent with

CURING IS COSTLY... PREVENTION PRICELESS!

SUPERVISOR EDMUND D. EDELMAN
FEBRUARY 6, 1978   Page 2

an acceptable radiograph for a dental x-ray examination. Generally, this
results not only in a substantial reduction in radiation but a corresponding
improvement in the quality of the dental radiograph.

In recent years, the law has been amended to require every x-ray technician
in a dental office to pass an examination in radiation safety permitting
them to operate dental radiographic equipment. This law has served to ex-
pand the quality of dental x-ray safety where x-ray is used. The typical
dental patient is the beneficiary of the increased knowledge and skills
gained by the dental x-ray operators who now deal more effectively with
protection of the patient.

A copy of that portion of the California Radiation Control Regulations
applicable to dental x-ray facilities is attached for your information.
The only limitations to the goal of optimum dental x-ray safety in the
community are those existing in the State law. However, periodic changes
in the law are adopted as needed to insure a continuing high safety level
in dental offices. The Radiation Management Office, in addition to its'
inspectional activity, routinely deals with a variety of public inquiries
and requests on all aspects of radiation safety.

MEC:JEK:mh

DEPARTMENT OF HEALTH SERVICES
714-744 P STREET
SACRAMENTO, CALIFORNIA 95814

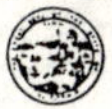

8 March 1979

SUBJECT: Dental X-ray Inspection Program

Dear Mr. Barmus

The State Controller's staff requested that I provide you with information relating to the State Department of Health Services program to regulate for safety X-ray machines in dental offices.

The Department is responsible for inspecting dental (and many other) X-ray machines to protect against unsafe levels of radiation. The program is self-supporting, paid for out of X-ray inspection fees imposed on the owners and operators, i.e., those licensed to apply X-rays, not by a broad general tax on the public.

The Department does have the legal right to cite violations and to require corrections of hazardous conditions involving X-ray machines. In fact the Department can also go to court to secure injunctions to prohibit the operation of unsafe X-ray equipment.

Pete Weisser
Information Officer
Department of Health Services
(916) 445-1967

UNITED STATES GENERAL ACCOUNTING OFFICE
WASHINGTON, D.C. 20548

HUMAN RESOURCES
DIVISION

JUN 1 3 1980

HRO-OTH-195

Dear Mr. Barmus

This is in response to your letter of May 20, 1980 to the Comptroller General of the United States.

We share your concern that Federal and State programs do not provide comprehensive protection from overexposure or unnecessary exposure to X-rays. Our report "Radiation Control Programs Provide Limited Protection", a copy of which is enclosed, discusses Federal and State radiation protection efforts.

Robert F. Hughes
Group Director

The Cancer Risk Nobody Dares to Talk About

DEPARTMENT OF HEALTH SERVICES
714/744 P STREET
SACRAMENTO, CA 95814
(916) 445-6256

April 3, 1979

Dear Mr. Barmus

Your letters regarding dental X-ray safety sent to Mr. Pete Weisser, dated March 17, 1979, and to Mr. Joseph Ward, dated March 21, 1979, have been forwarded to me for reply.

I believe there was a misunderstanding of your question, or of our answer, regarding jurisdiction over the use of X-rays by dentists. Our Department does not have jurisdiction over the competence and certification of dentists or their employees to perform dental radiography. This is the responsibility of the State Board of Dental Examiners in the Department of Consumer Affairs. Our Department does, however, have the responsibility for the safety of dental X-ray equipment and its use.

There is no specific legal restriction on the radiation exposure to the patient per dental X-ray film. The minimum exposure achievable on dental X-ray equipment commonly ranges from 100 mR to 500 mR per film, depending on the type of equipment used, and certain exposure factors such as kilovolts, cone length, beam quality, etc.

Electronic timers are not required and are not necessary to achieve a high quality radiograph with minimum patient exposure. Consistency or "repeatibility" is the most important quality of the dental X-ray timer. A mechanical timer can require more elapsed time to function consistently but this can be compensated for by adjusting the milliamperes or cone length or other factor to provide a safe, low exposure per film.

A California regulation requiring shielded open-ended cones or cylinders (Section 30311(d)(2) of the California Radiation Control Regulations) became effective for new equipment on September 1, 1978. However, the Federal Bureau of Radiological Health, from whom we get many of our California standards, recently recommended against this requirement because of questionable safety value, and we are now in the process of dropping this requirement.

Mechanical film-holding devices require that extra materials be placed in the patients' mouth to hold the film. This is a discomfort and sometimes a cause for alarm to some patients. Mainly for these reasons, I believe, the

-2-   April 3, 1979

National Council on Radiation Protection and Measurements (NCRP), which is the primary source for our X-ray standards, has not made mechanical film holders a high-priority safety item. When a patient holds a film in his mouth with his hand the radiation damage to the patient is very probably less than when he doesn't use his hand. This is because his hand absorbs some of the radiation which would have otherwise been absorbed by the more radiosensitive tissues on the far side of the mouth and head.

We keep information on the safety inspections we make of all dental installations. If you wish specific information on the safety findings of one or a few dentists, we can provide this as allowed under the public information rules. We do not tabulate and publish data on inspection findings of individuals since this is very costly and time-consuming and is beyond the scope of our budget and program.

The United States Department of Health, Education, and Welfare made a very comprehensive study of all types of X-ray uses in the healing arts in 1970 throughout the United States, and has published its findings in several publications. One of these is "Population Exposure to X-rays, United States, 1970", DHEW Publication (FDA) 73-8047, and is for sale by the United States Government Printing Office, Washington, D. C. 20402.

Section 30311 of the California Radiation Control Regulations contains our special regulations covering the use of X-rays in dentistry. We routinely inspect for compliance with these regulations. At the present time we do not have regulations covering many factors which closely affect the patient exposure such as film speed, film processing techniques, minimum kV, exposure factors and maximum allowable patient exposure per film.

Our current practice is to make recommendations to the dentist to correct any of these factors when found faulty. Many dentists follow our recommendations and we are able to achieve substantial exposure reductions. The cases of high patient exposure you described during our discussion were obviously where our recommendations were not followed.

For reasons of uniformity and for general acceptance, our regulations on X-ray safety are nearly always copied from national standards such as those of the NCRP or the Federal Bureau of Radiological Health. We are very hesitant to adopt new regulations on film processing, maximum patient exposure, etc. unless they are promulgated by agencies such as these.

I hope the above discussion plus our telephone conversation of yesterday have answered your questions. Please let me know if you have others.

Sincerely,

Robert England, Supervisor
X-radiation Control Unit
Radiologic Health Section

<u>EXCERPTS</u>

HEW Publication (FDA) 76-8042

DENTAL EXPOSURE
NORMALIZATION TECHNIQUE
"DENT"
INSTRUCTION MANUAL

<u>Background</u>

Studies of intraoral x-ray examinations have shown exposures at the skin ranging from 100 to over 5,000 mR per film. Consequently, a study was conducted by the Bureau of Radiological Health to empirically determine the exposures required for quality dental radiographs.

Acceptable X-ray Exposure Ranges

kVp	mm Al	Approx. mR/film
50	1.5	400-550
65	1.5	300-450
75	2.5	200-325
90	2.5	100-200

<u>Exposure Readings Outside the Acceptable Exposure Ranges</u>

Once the exposed TLD chips have been read, transfer the calculated mR/film to the master record sheet. Examine each reading to determine if the machine output per film exceeds the upper limit of the exposure range at the reported kilovoltage (see graph below, Acceptable X-Ray Exposure Ranges). Flag those readings which are outside the acceptable ranges. Machines with readings that fall below the range for the reported kilovoltage are also suspect, requiring either a repeat of the exposure card procedure or a scheduled office visit.

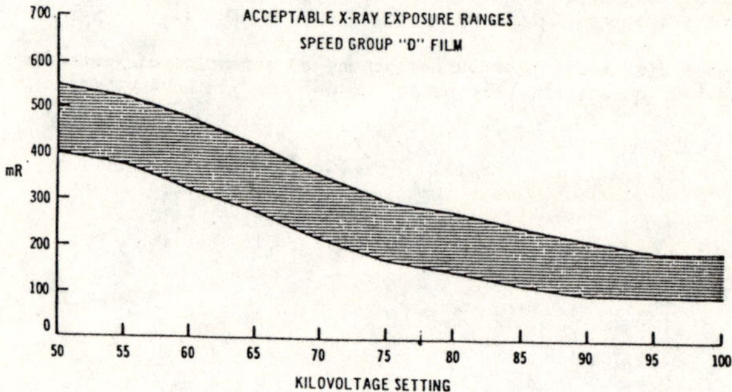

DEPARTMENT OF HEALTH SERVICES
714/744 P STREET
SACRAMENTO, CA 95814

(916) 445-6256

January 21, 1981

Pursuant to your most recent letter, our X-ray machine registration process
does not require the purchaser of an X-ray machine to inform the department
about HEW certification of his or her equipment.

For this reason, we are unable to answer your question as to how many or
which machines   are HEW certified.

Sincerely,

Suzanne Ritter
Senior Health Physicist
X-radiation Control Unit
Radiologic Health Section

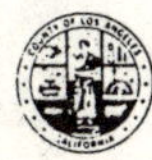

COUNTY OF LOS ANGELES • DEPARTMENT OF HEALTH SERVICES

313 NORTH FIGUEROA STREET • LOS ANGELES, CALIFORNIA 90012 • (213) 974- 7891

June 2, 1982

Thank you for your letter of May 19, 1982 addressed to Kathleen
Kaufman of our staff inquiring about certified x-ray equipment.

Although as much as twenty percent of all x-ray machines in use in
the County of Los Angeles are certified as meeting Federal Performance Standards, we do not have a breakdown of the location of the
certified units. If you have a specific facility in mind, we may
be able to verify if a certified machine is located there.

I am sorry we cannot provide the information you requested, however,
your concern about radiation safety is most appreciated.

Sincerely,

Joseph E. Karbus, Director
Occupational Health & Radiation Management

JEK:w

THE CANCER RISK NOBODY DARES TO TALK ABOUT

A STUDY OF THE NEED FOR CONTROLLING THE SALE OF ANTIQUATED
X-RAY EQUIPMENT

INTRODUCTION

Background

Since 1959 the United States Public Health Service has been assisting States in the development of X-ray control programs. These programs have been directed at the registration and correction of deficiencies on X-ray equipment so that it meets the requirement of either the State radiation protection code or the recommendations of the National Council on Radiation Protection and Measurements.

The Radiation Control for Health and Safety Act of 1968, P.L. 90-602, directs the Secretary of Health, Education, and Welfare to develop and administer performance standards to control the emission of electronic product radiation; however, any such standards promulgated under the act would be applicable only to those electronic products manufactured after the effective date of the standard.

The Congress has directed the Secretary to conduct studies to determine any gaps and inconsistencies in the present controls. Further, the Secretary is required to make a report or reports to the Congress on or before January 1, 1970 and from time to time therafter as he may find necessary together with such recommendations for legislation as he may deem appropriate. This report was prepared in partial fulfillment of the Secretary's responsibilities under Section 357 of the act.

DEPARTMENT OF HEALTH & HUMAN SERVICES   Public Health Service

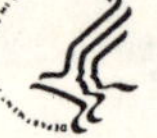

Food and Drug Administration
Rockville MD 20857

July 2, 1981

I have your letter of June 25, 1981, acknowledging receipt of the

study of "Antiquated X-ray Equipment," mandated by Section 357 of

the Radiation Control for Health and Safety Act of 1968. The study,

which was carried out by the Bureau of Radiological Health, became

in effect the Secretary's report to the Congress. There was no

additional document. The conclusions and recommendations that resulted

from the study, which comprised the substance of the study's findings,

were incorporated into the copy of the report you received.

Sincerely yours,

J. Arthur Lazell
Assistant Director
Bureau of Radiological Health

NOTES

1. U.S. Senate Report No. 1432, *Radiation Control for Health and Safety Act of 1968*, "Legislative History," page 4314.

2. Ibid, page. 4315.

3. Legislative Analyst's report to Art Torres, Chairman, Assembly Health and Welfare Committee, concerning x-ray inspections, November 23, 1981.

4. Department of Health, Education, and Welfare (HEW) publication (FDA) 78-8050, *A Practitioner's Guide to The Diagnostic X-Ray Equipment Standard*, February 1978.

5. Arthur C. Upton, M.D., Director, National Cancer Institute, Statement on "Carcinogenic Hazards of Low-Level Radiation," before the Subcommittee on Health and the Environment, February 8 and 9, 1978.

6. "Lung Cancer Now Deadliest Form for California Women," *Los Angeles Times*, October 14, 1983.

7. "A Plague of Sunshine," *Prevention*, July 1983.

8. "Thyroid Cancer," *Western Journal of Medicine*, November 1979.

9. "Her Most Serious Medical Problem," *Los Angeles Times*, December 5, 1982.

10. "Breast Cancer — A Disease of the Rich," *Los Angeles Times*, February 6, 1983.

11. *Cancer in China*, Report on the American Cancer Delegation's visit to the People's Republic of China, 1977.

12. Donald Kennedy, Commissioner, Food and Drug Administration, Public Health Service, Department of Health, Education, and Welfare; Statement before the Subcommittee on Health and the Environment, July 12, 1978.

13. Comptroller General of the United States, report entitled *Radiation Control Programs Provide Limited Protection*, December 4, 1979.

14. (FDA) 80-8111, *Get the Picture on . . . Dental X-Rays*.

15. DHEW Publication No. (NIH) 79-1621, 1979, *Progress Against Breast Cancer, What You Can Do About It.*

16. "That Costly Physical," *Consumer Reports,* October 1980.

17. Phil Donahue TV Show, June 21, 1983.

18. *Federal Performance Standard for Diagnostic X-Ray Systems Code of Federal Regulations,* Title 21, Section 1020.30 through 1020.32.

19. Alice Dolezal, Section of Radiation Control, Minnesota Department of Health, *What Can And Needs To Be Done By State/Local Radiation Control Agencies,* 9th Annual National Conference on Radiation Control, June 19-23, 1977, published by U.S. Department of Health, Education, and Welfare (FDA).

20. Jerre E. Jensen, R.T.; Priscilla F. Butler, M.S.; Rockville, Maryland, *Breast Exposure: Nationwide Trends; A Mammography Quality Assurance Program — Results To Date.* American Society of Radiologic Technologists, Vol. 50, No. 3, 1978.

21. Letter from the Department of Health Services, Sacramento, California, dated April 26, 1979.

22. Priscilla W. Laws, Ph.D., and Ralph Nader's Public Citizen Health Research Group, *The X-Ray Information Book,* published by Farrar, Straus & Giroux in 1983.

23. "Order More Diagnostic Tests," *Medical Economics,* September 30, 1974.

24. State of California, Department of Consumer Affairs, Board of Dental Examiners, *Radiation Protection in Dental Practice.*

25. A. B. Reiskin, Professor of Radiology, Department of Oral Diagnosis, School of Dental Medicine, University of Connecticut. Statement before the Subcommittee on Health and the Environment, of the Committee on Interstate and Foreign Commerce, July 11, 1978.

26. State of California, Department of Health Services, Sacramento, California, "California Radiation Control Regulations," *California Administrative Code,* Title 17, Health.

27. HEW Publication (FDA) 76-8042, *Dental Exposure Normalization Technique "DENT" Instruction Manual.*

28. KABC-TV 7, Los Angeles, California, May 10-14, 1982.

29. "What the federal X-ray regulations mean to the dentist," *Journal of the American Dental Association* (JADA), October 1977.

30. "Self-Regulation vs. Government Intervention," *Journal of the American Dental Association,* September 1981.

31. H.R. 672, H.R. 1526, H.R. 9125; bills of the 93rd Congress (1973-1974).

Notes

32. "Letters to the Editor," *The Journal of the American Dental Association,* December 1979, Volume 99, No. 6.
33. "Danger Is Negligible in Dental X-Rays," *Los Angeles Times,* March 6, 1978.
34. "Glamour Medical Report," *Glamour,* March 1979.
35. "The new worry over x-rays and what you can do about it," *Good Housekeeping,* July 1979.
36. "X-Ray . . . How Often? How Safe?" *Mademoiselle,* December 1980.
37. HEW Publication (FDA) 77-8013, *The Mean Active Bone Marrow Dose to the Adult Population of the United States from Diagnostic Radiology.*
38. P.L. 90-602, Section 357, *The Radiation Control for Health and Safety Act of 1968.*

INDEX